Acclaim for *Dr. Attwood's Low-*

"If we are at all serious about prolonging life and lowering our death rates, the place to start is not after these lethal diseases strike, in middle or old age, but by studying Dr. Attwood's book and implementing his suggestions when our children are young. His work is thorough, clear, and persuasive."
—Dr. Benjamin Spock

"Hurray! At last, a pediatrician willing to provide parents with advice on the best possible diet for their children."
—Michael Jacobson, Ph.D., Center for Science in the Public Interest

"Dr. Attwood has set a standard for childhood nutrition that is without peer. His message is bold, reliable, and forward-looking. This book ought to be on every pediatrician's shelf. It could become a classic."
—T. Colin Campbell, Ph.D., Jacob Gould Schurman Professor of Nutritional Biochemistry, Cornell University, and director of the China Health Project

"Magnificent. I couldn't put this book down. It is not only well researched, it's well written and contains useful material for everybody—especially parents, who will find ways to feed their kids correctly."
—Frank A. Oski, M.D., Given Professor of Pediatrics and chairman of the Department of Pediatrics, Johns Hopkins University, and editor in chief of the standard textbook *Principles and Practice of Pediatrics*

"Makes an insightful and eloquent statement to parents that proper nutrition is, indeed, the best medicine that you can give your children, and that their future health depends on it. In fact, nutritional medicine is the medicine of the twenty-first century."
—Dr. Art Mollen, syndicated health columnist and author of *The Anti-Aging Diet*

"Best nutrition book in fifty years. It is scientifically based, and written in a style that is easy to read and understand. The focus is on children's nutrition, but the message will have a positive impact on all family members."
—E. Leslie Knight, Ph.D., F.A.C.S.M., director of the national seminars "The Role of Nutrition and Exercise in Preventive Medicine"

"Sends an important message to parents: a healthy body tomorrow begins with a healthy diet today—in childhood. *But current dietary recommendations for children are obsolete.* Dr. Attwood spells out an alternative nutrition strategy that is sensible and progressive. Every concerned parent should read this book."
—Suzanne Havala, M.S., R.D., L.D.N., primary author, "Position of the American Dietetic Association: Vegetarian Diets"

"This book will emerge as a classic. It will set the standard for generations to come. 'Must' reading for every pediatrician, parent, nutritionist, public policy planner, and anyone who touches the lives of children."
—Dr. Hans Diehl, cardiovascular epidemiologist and director of the Lifestyle Medicine Institute

"A well-researched, practical guide for parents and an invaluable resource for pediatricians as well. When we invest in better foods for our children, the payoff is a lifetime of good health and productivity. Dr. Attwood shows how to go about it."
—Neal D. Barnard, M.D., president, Physicians Committee for Responsible Medicine

"To have your child grow up healthy into adolescence and beyond, Dr. Attwood's book gives you precisely the right prescription. All you have to do is follow it."
—Ernst L. Wynder, M.D., president, American Health Foundation

PENGUIN BOOKS

DR. ATTWOOD'S LOW–FAT PRESCRIPTION FOR KIDS

Charles R. Attwood, M.D., F.A.A.P., directs one of the nation's largest solo pediatric private practices, with a primary emphasis on preventive medicine and children's nutrition, and writes frequently for various medical publications. His seminars have been presented to physicians, dieticians, educators, and parents throughout the nation. He lives with his wife, Jo Anna, in Crowley, Louisiana.

Dr. Attwood's

Low-Fat Prescription for Kids

Charles R. Attwood, M.D.

PENGUIN BOOKS

PENGUIN BOOKS
Published by the Penguin Group
Penguin Books USA Inc., 375 Hudson Street, New York, New York 10014, U.S.A.
Penguin Books Ltd, 27 Wrights Lane, London W8 5TZ, England
Penguin Books Australia Ltd, Ringwood, Victoria, Australia
Penguin Books Canada Ltd, 10 Alcorn Avenue, Toronto, Ontario, Canada M4V 3B2
Penguin Books (N.Z.) Ltd, 182–190 Wairau Road, Auckland 10, New Zealand

Penguin Books Ltd, Registered Offices: Harmondsworth, Middlesex, England

First published in the United States of America by Viking Penguin,
a division of Penguin Books USA Inc., 1995
Published in Penguin Books 1996

1 3 5 7 9 10 8 6 4 2

The recipes in this book have been analyzed by the Diet Modification Clinic
at Baylor College of Medicine in Houston, Texas.

A NOTE TO THE READER
The ideas, procedures, and suggestions contained in this book are not
intended as a substitute for consulting with your physician.
All matters regarding your health require medical supervision.

THE LIBRARY OF CONGRESS HAS CATALOGUED THE HARDCOVER AS FOLLOWS:
Attwood, Charles R.
Dr. Attwood's low-fat prescription for kids:
a pediatrician's program of preventive nutrition/Charles R. Attwood.
p.   cm.
Includes index.
ISBN 0-670-85829-3 (hc.)
ISBN 0 14 02.3644 9 (pbk.)
1. Children—Nutrition.   2. Low-fat diet.   I. Title.
RJ206.A87   1995
613.2´8—dc20   94–20258

Printed in the United States of America
Set in Garamond Light
Designed by Victoria Hartman

Dedicated to
Kathy, Mary, Laura,
and Paul

We owe our children a set of good habits; for habit is to be their best friend or their worst enemy, not only during childhood, but through all the years. We shall therefore need to repeat every now and then nature's irrevocable law: that back of every habit lies a series of acts; that ahead of every act lies a habit; that a habit is nine tenths of conduct; that conduct is but character in the making; and that character ends in destiny.

—*George Herbert Betts*
Educator, University of Chicago
(1868–1934)

Foreword

*T*his book's message is that the only way to combat our country's shockingly high death rates for coronary heart disease, stroke, and cancer in adulthood is to adopt a low-fat diet beginning in childhood. But before I discuss the author's position, let me tell you a little about his unique background.

Dr. Charles Attwood is a pediatrician of unusually broad and progressive interests. In the 30 years between finishing his medical training and writing this pioneering book, he built a large practice in Crowley, Louisiana, where he still works.

He once wrote a series of 10 articles for the journal *Medical Economics* on how he developed such a large, loyal practice in the middle of Cajun country. He told how he sometimes takes the initiative in telephoning the parents when a child has been sick and he hasn't heard from them about the child's progress, a thoughtful and unfamiliar attention. Several times a year, he sits down with his office staff and six or eight parents for a frank and informal conversation, perhaps over lunch, about what is unsatisfactory and what is pleasing about his services and those of the staff. (Other physicians too have observed that parents speak much more freely in a group.) His receptionist tries to get the same sort of feedback from parents after each visit by asking, "How did things go today?" As might be expected, the most common complaint over the years was about waiting time, until doctor and staff came up with a variety of ingenious solutions to delays, including an electric wall-board that tells the nurses what the patient in each examining room needs, such as a particular vaccine.

I admire particularly Dr. Attwood's article that frankly disagrees with those physicians who refuse to see patients whose bills will be paid by Medicaid, claiming that the fee schedule is too low, or that there is too long a delay in payment, or that such patients' scruffiness drives other patients away from the office.

In his younger years, he was a marathon runner; this may account at least in part for his long-standing interest in physical exercise and health, one result of which is his strong emphasis on preventive medicine in his pediatric practice.

For a number of years now, Dr. Attwood has been concerned with the high incidence of death by coronary heart disease and also by stroke and cancer. Coronary disease is the gradual plugging of the coronary arteries, which supply blood to the muscles of the heart, with "plaques" of fat and calcium in the walls of these arteries. It is now by far the most common cause of death in our country. Most of the deaths occur in middle or old age. But the evidence has been accumulating for years—from the examination of the hearts of children and young people who have died in accidents—that the process of gradual blocking of the coronary arteries begins not in adulthood but in childhood, even as young as the preschool years; and also that the main cause of this arteriosclerosis ("hardening of the arteries") is the steadily increasing amount of fat in the American diet, particularly "saturated" animal fats such as those found in meat, chicken, milk, and cheeses. If there was another disease that caused half a million deaths a year, you can be sure that the public would be acutely aware of the danger, and that the cure or prevention would be practiced universally. Why, then, is arteriosclerosis's extreme danger to life accepted so casually, and why are the measures needed to prevent it so regularly ignored?

One explanation is that there is a long gap, usually about half a century, between childhood, when the American high-fat diet is established (without any hints that it might be lethal—in fact, it's what everyone in the family is happily eating), and middle or old age, when the consequences suddenly show up—a first heart attack. At that point, after years of consuming cholesterol and fat-laden foods, many people are instructed to change to low-fat diets.

But studies have shown how difficult it is for people in any society to give up their familiar diets and to accept different ones. That's why Americans find it so difficult, if not impossible, to take the warning that they should give up the foods they've relished all their lives without any noticeable ill effects—hamburgers, steaks, poultry, French fries, potato chips, eggs, bacon, butter, cheese, cream, cream sauces, ice cream, and whole milk.

Following the logic of these various truths, Dr. Attwood comes to the only possible conclusion: that the way to reverse our tragic death rates in adulthood is for parents to stop teaching their children to love and demand today's high-fat diet. (Babies in the first year or two need preferably breast milk or commercially prepared baby formula that has been modified to be more like breast milk and is fairly high in fat.) So, if we are at all serious about prolonging life and lowering our high death rates, the place to start is not after these lethal diseases strike, in middle or old age, but by studying Dr. Attwood's book and implementing his suggestions when our children are young. His work is thorough, clear, and persuasive.

Part One of this book will prove most valuable to parents. Here Dr. Attwood demolishes 12 common myths that deny the urgency of reducing the swollen amounts of fat in the present American diet—myths that are cherished by many parents (and some physicians and nutritionists). These include the myth that it is not really necessary to be concerned with cholesterol levels in the early years of a child's life, and the myth that such a diet would cause nutritional deficiencies or growth retardation.

Part Two offers a lot of practical advice, including how to make this diet more acceptable to children by introducing it in a series of 4 stages; how to deal with eating out; what to do about school; and how to become a low-fat shopper at the supermarket.

Part Three presents the scientific underpinnings of a low-fat diet; and Part Four contains helpful hints from a mother's point of view, including children-tested menus and recipes.

I identify with the book's purpose, because I was raised on a vegetarian diet until the age of 12, became 6 feet 4 inches tall by 14, rowed on an 8-oared crew that won gold medals in the 1924 Olympics, became a pediatrician because pediatrics is primarily preventive, then went back to a low-fat diet at 88 because of a transient stroke—and am now doing fine at 91!

—*Dr. Benjamin Spock*

Acknowledgments

I wish to express my sincerest gratitude to the following people, who helped make this book possible. With their constant ideas and encouragement I was finally able to stop writing at the end of the tenth draft.

My wife, Jo Anna, who has sat beside me at dozens of scientific conferences and medical meetings over the years, has never taken a passive role. Her questions, opinions, and suggestions have been helpful and supportive.

Warren La Coste, my friend and regular Thursday-evening "sounding board," was the first to encourage me to set aside my magazine-essay projects and to begin writing this book. His pep talks continued throughout the 3-year project.

Patti Breitman, my literary agent, guided the book through its early proposal stages and continued to offer wonderful suggestions until I turned in the final manuscript.

Mindy Werner, my editor at Viking, worked over each new re-write with her No. 2 pencil until the manuscript finally said what we had in mind. Her editorial magic will be appreciated as you read.

Victoria Moran, author of *Get the Fat Out*, who also wrote the essay "A Mom's Guide to Happy, Low-Fat Kids" for this book, was the first to say "wonderful" when she read my first rough copy.

Sonnet Pierce complemented the final section of the book with her original, children-tested, low-fat recipes.

My new friends Dr. Benjamin Spock and his wife, Mary Morgan, spent many hours reading my manuscript while their many other projects lay waiting. Their help was invaluable.

For their ideas, research, suggestions, and encouragement at our meetings at conferences through the years, I wish to thank Dr. Gerald Berenson, Dr. Neal Barnard, Dr. T. Colin Campbell, Dr. William Castelli, Dr. Peter Jones, Dr. Hans Diehl, Dr. Caldwell B. Esselstyn, Jr., Dr. Dean Ornish, Dr. Peter Wood, Dr. Les Knight, and Dr. Ernst Wynder. Lynne Scott, at the Diet Modification Clinic at Baylor College of Medicine in Houston, Texas, did the ingredient analysis for the recipes.

My clinic staff, who helped me carry on a busy practice while I was totally focused on writing this book, made it possible to do both. My sincere thanks go to JoAnn Murrin, Billie Corman, Ramona Stein, Pam Dailey, Kara Miller, Faye Perry, Janet Ellingson, Lee Ellingson, Deanna Treadway, Agnes Collins, Ronda Prather, Gail Johnson, and Jary Bullock.

And, finally, to the National Institutes of Health, the American Heart Association, and the American Academy of Pediatrics (of which I am a fellow), I express sincere appreciation for the research, education, and professional help they have provided over the many years of my medical practice. Despite our differences about dietary fat and cholesterol screening of children, expressed in this book, I have a great admiration for each of these organizations for their valuable contributions to the health and welfare of all Americans.

Contents

Foreword, by Dr. Benjamin Spock   vii

Acknowledgments   xi

Author's Note   xvii

Introduction: You Make the Rules   xix

Part One

Twelve Common Myths
About Low-Fat Diets for Children

Chapter 1. Myth One:
Controlling Cholesterol Can Wait   3

Chapter 2. Myth Two:
Controlling Obesity Can Wait   21

Chapter 3. Myth Three:
The "Fat Taste" Is Natural and Inborn   36

Chapter 4. Myth Four:
Small Reductions in Fat Will Do   41

Chapter 5. Myth Five:
Children's Diets Are Getting Better   50

Chapter 6. Myth Six:
Meat Is Needed for Protein and Iron   55

Chapter 7. Myth Seven:
Milk Is Needed for Calcium and Protein   62

Chapter 8. Myth Eight:
Low-Fat Diets Lack Vitamins and Minerals   70

Chapter 9. Myth Nine:
A Low-Fat Diet Means Limited Choices   78

Chapter 10. Myth Ten:
Low-Fat Diets Retard Growth   83

Chapter 11. Myth Eleven:
It's Obvious Which Foods Are High in Fat   89

Chapter 12. Myth Twelve:
No One Knows What's *Really* Best for My Child   95

Part Two
_____

Feeding Children in the Real World:
Practical Approaches

Chapter 13: 4 Stages to an Ideal Diet   101

Chapter 14: A Low-Fat Shopping Primer   110

Chapter 15: Back Home, Getting Started   128

Chapter 16: When Children Eat Out   133

Chapter 17: School Lunch Programs   139

Part Three
_____

So You Want Proof?
The Scientific Basis

Chapter 18: The Childhood Beginnings of Heart Disease   153

Chapter 19: Summit in the Desert   172

Chapter 20: How You're Misinformed   181

Part Four
_____

Helpful Hints, Menus,
and Children-Tested Recipes

Chapter 21: A Mom's Guide to Happy, Low-Fat Kids   197
by Victoria Moran

Chapter 22: Suggested Menus   217
by Victoria Moran

Chapter 23: Children-Tested Recipes   222
by Sonnet Pierce

Notes   253

Recommended Reading   271

Index   274

Author's Note

*T*he recommendations presented in this book are based on observations made during 32 years of pediatric practice and personal communication with dozens of scientific researchers in the fields of nutrition and preventive medicine. The suggestions and guidelines are appropriate for the overwhelming majority of children over the age of 2; however, since each individual child may have unique medical needs, I strongly recommend that you adopt my diet suggestions with the approval of your child's personal physician.

The word "diet," used throughout the book, doesn't refer to short-term eating changes—with a clear beginning and a much-awaited ending—so commonly recommended in "diet books." The confused reader has my sympathy, because those books share shelf space with books such as mine, where the word "diet" means a permanent life-style program or a way of life. Reports of scientific studies, conferences, and medical-journal articles generally use the word "diet" in this context. "Westernized diet" refers to the typical eating habits in America and most other industrialized nations.

Introduction:
You Make the Rules

There is nothing as powerful
as an idea whose time has come
— *Victor Hugo*
(1802–85)

*S*everal years ago, while explaining to a group of elementary-school students what effect their diets may have upon their health, I was sadly aware that, without a considerable reduction in their dietary fat, from dairy products, meat, and oils, most of them would not live out their full life spans. If they were to have a thirtieth class reunion, the majority would already have unrecognized heart disease or cancer poised to strike during their most productive and pleasurable years.

The first changes of coronary heart disease, fatty deposits in the coronary arteries, begin appearing by age 3 in children eating a typical American diet. By age 12 nearly 70 percent of children are affected—and more advanced deposits rapidly appear throughout the teens. These early stages of the disease are found in virtually all young adults by the age of 21.

As you will read later in Chapter 18, these stunning facts have been documented conclusively by clinical and autopsy studies conducted during the past four decades. These same studies also show that this potentially fatal disease may be prevented by simple dietary changes.

Dr. Lloyd Kolbe, director of adolescent and school health of the Centers for Disease Control and Prevention, told pediatricians at the 1993 annual meeting of the American Academy of Pediatrics that the major health problems confronting our nation today are caused, in large part, by behaviors established during youth. The greatest health risks for today's children, he said, are those of heart disease and cancer as adults. Dr. Kolbe was expressing one of the most serious challenges facing parents, physicians, and school health officials today. Such diseases, responsible for half of all adult deaths, he feels, are not an inevitable part of growing older. Both are related to a child's diet.

The most deadly of these—and the most preventable—is coronary heart disease, which is caused by a blockage by cholesterol deposits within the coronary arteries, therefore interfering with the supply of oxygen and vital nutrients to the heart muscle itself. *The fact is, 1.5 million adults will have heart attacks each year—and 500,000 of them will die. Three out of 5 of this half-million will die suddenly, without sufficient time to reach a hospital. More will die of the disease months or years later, after an indefinite period of chronic disability. Once this disease is established, there is no real cure.*

The late Dr. John Knowles, while president of the Rockefeller Foundation, wrote that 99 percent of us are born healthy and are made sick as a result of personal misbehavior or environmental conditions. He suggested that the ability to lengthen one's life depends first on the capacity not to shorten it.

The first place we should look for life-shortening behaviors is the eating habits of our children. Most people are surprised to learn just how many of our adult diseases are related to what we eat throughout our early and middle years. Of the 10 leading causes of death in the United States (heart disease, cancer, stroke, emphysema, accidents, pneumonia, diabetes, suicide, AIDS, and homicide), only three are *not* related to what we eat or drink, including alcohol. These are emphysema (related to smoking), pneumonia, and AIDS.

Physicians, like myself, who practice preventive medicine believe that more than 95 percent of coronary-artery disease can be prevented by meaningful reductions in dietary fat if implemented early in life. This conclusion is based on the near absence of this disease in areas of the world (rural China, South America, and eastern Africa) where a very low-fat diet is consumed throughout life. On the other hand, children who consume a typical American high-fat diet have elevated blood-cholesterol levels and fatty deposits within their arteries at an early age.

In the United States, among adults—*even those who have reduced their fat intake moderately*—coronary heart disease remains the number-one cause of death. This includes the first baby boomers, who grew up on a high-fat diet and are now reaching their fiftieth birthday. Furthermore, Chinese immigrants who have spent their childhood in the United States, consuming the typical high-fat diet, and their peers who have emigrated to Asian cities but adopted the "Americanized diet," have the same high rate of heart disease as native-born Americans. *This takes only one generation when the high-fat diets begin during childhood.*

Coronary-artery disease is not the only risk for children consuming excessive dietary fat. The National Cancer Institute (NCI) estimates that at least 35 percent of all cancers are linked to food. This relationship to food—usually excess dietary fat—may be more common than the NCI suspects, according to a 1992 report issued by the National Academy of Sciences. In the publication *Eat for Life*, the Academy's Committee on Diet and Health points out that we simply do not know how much cancer is food-related but that estimates among researchers range up to 70 percent.

There is reason to suspect that victims of either cancer or heart disease are afflicted with these maladies in part because of *what they ate during their childhood.* Among all countries of the world where records are kept, countries in which children's diets are high in fat record a high rate of heart disease and cancer deaths. These children who later develop heart disease or cancer as adults have been found to eat excess dietary fat and consume few fresh vegetables, fruits, and grains (complex carbohydrates). This risk may be extended when the fat habit persists throughout adulthood; however, the greatest peril exists when this eating pattern is established

during the growing years. Lifetime eating habits are usually established by the age of 8.

Among all cancers, those of the prostate and breast may be the
most likely to stem from children's eating habits. Prostate cancer,
even though only diagnosed in the elderly, has been found to be
related to diets high in animal fat. The disease is rare in developing
countries, where little fat is eaten throughout life, whereas the highest rates are among elderly men in the United States and England
who have typically been meat-eaters since childhood. On the other
hand, *Seventh-Day Adventists raised as vegetarians have lower rates
of prostate cancer during their later years than those who become
vegetarians later in life.*

Breast cancer is less common among women who ate little or no
meat during childhood. Supporting this conclusion is the fact that
there is very little breast cancer among Asians—except those who
grew up in Western nations, where they consumed the typical high-
fat diet. Japanese women who emigrated from their homeland to
the United States and have adopted a Western diet as adults maintain their low risk for breast cancer. *It is the second generation,
their daughters, who, on a typical high-fat American diet, have an
increased incidence of breast cancer, many times that of their cous-
ins who grew up in rural Japan.*

Similarly, another study has shown that Scottish women, whose
childhood was essentially meatless and dairyless during World War
II (when they ate mostly fresh vegetables and whole-grain bread),
were found to have much less breast cancer than expected during
their premenopausal years, *even though they consumed a typical
Western diet as adults.* The author of this study, Dr. Peter Boyle—
now Director of the Division of Epidemiology and Biostatistics at
the Instituto Europeo di Oncologia in Milan, Italy—suggested in his
1987 report that some unknown factor was protecting these women.
Since then, he and other researchers have concluded that *the* "unknown" protective factor was probably their lack of meat and dairy
products during childhood.

Consuming a very low-fat diet during childhood is known to result in a later onset of menstruation—in rural Chinese and Japanese
girls, to the age of 16 to 18. This *lessens* the lifetime risk of breast

cancer, suggests Dr. Hans Diehl of the Lifestyle Medicine Institute in Loma Linda, California, because the breast tissue undergoes fewer years of estrogen exposure.

Another explanation was suggested to me by Dr. John Weisburger, a scientist at the American Health Foundation. There is evidence that changes later leading to cancer may appear in the breast tissue at times of greater cell reproduction and tissue growth, such as around the time of puberty. A high-fat diet at this time may be more carcinogenic than it would be later on in life. This has proved true for other cancer-producing agents. For example, the single pulse of radiation at the time of the Hiroshima nuclear explosion led to a risk of later breast cancer four times greater among girls 10 to 19 years old than among adult women.

The relationship of breast cancer to fat in the *adult* diet is less clear. A Harvard study by Dr. Walter Willett found little change in the risk of breast cancer among women placed on a *moderately* low-fat diet (in which 30 percent of the calories consumed come from fat) for up to eight years. These women ate a typical high-fat American diet during their childhood, and their fat consumption was reduced for a few years as adults. No women were knowingly included in the study who had consumed a low-fat diet since childhood. Meanwhile, the Italian study described below may have shown a relationship of dietary fat during childhood to adult breast cancer.

A report in the *Journal of the National Cancer Institute* compared Italian women in whose diet 36 percent of the calories came from fat to those who consumed less than 28 percent fat. The higher-fat group had *three times* the breast-cancer risk of the lower-fat women. However, this was not an intervention study like the one done at Harvard, where the experimenters reduced the fat in subjects' diet for eight years. *These Italian women eating less than 28 percent of calories from fat were selected at random from an area in northern Italy where individuals have generally consumed a low-fat diet from childhood.* This suggests either that the adult fat consumption must be less than 28 percent of calories to prevent breast cancer or that the women's diet during childhood was protective. I suspect that both factors are important.

Our Inadequate "Official" Guidelines

The cancer-diet relationship is convincing at the least, but there can be no doubt about the role played by dietary fat in coronary heart disease. Our nation's number one killer claims a life every 34 seconds—men and women in approximately equal numbers. It costs the nation more than $100 billion annually, yet it can be prevented for a tiny fraction of this amount. Consuming a diet in which fat constitutes only 10–15 percent of calories, starting in childhood, practically eliminates the risk of coronary-artery disease, except for individuals with rare genetic disorders, and reduces the risk of strokes, hypertension, diabetes, and many cancers. Virtually no one questions this. So why is it that the National Institutes of Health (NIH) and private research foundations commit barely 1–3 percent of their total funding to encourage *any* degree of change in the American diet? Even less is being done to eliminate the fat habit in children. American Heart Association (AHA) President Suzanne Oparil said to a group of doctors in New Orleans in 1994 that almost none of NIH's grant money is devoted to children's diet research and only 6 cents of every federal dollar is spent on childhood and youth programs of *any* kind.

The late Dr. Denis Burkitt, famed proponent of dietary fiber, illustrated with a metaphor this misplaced emphasis of the *treatment approach* by Western medicine:

> If people are falling over the edge of a cliff and sustaining injuries, the problem could be dealt with by stationing ambulances at the bottom or erecting a fence at the top. Unfortunately, we put far too much effort into the positioning of ambulances and far too little into the simple approach of erecting fences.

In Dr. Burkitt's example, the enormously expensive use of angioplasty, bypass surgery, and high-tech coronary-care units might be sympolized by the use of helicoptors to assist the ambulances at the bottom of the cliff. The sensible, inexpensive, and far more effective way to *prevent* people from metaphorically falling over the cliff is to embrace the nutritional changes recommended in this book, symbolized by the fence.

The First National Cholesterol Conference, held in 1988 in Washington, D.C., by the NIH, left me with mixed feelings. Guidelines had finally been set by their newly organized National Cholesterol Education Program (NCEP), with the sole purpose of preventing coronary-artery disease. Unfortunately, the guidelines were for adults only, and the recommended reductions of dietary fat—up to 30 percent of calories from fat, among which 10 percent are from saturated fat—were not based on proven scientific data, but on what the NIH *thought* the public would accept. Members of the NCEP committee admitted their fear that recommendations of further fat reductions, even though scientifically indicated, would be intimidating, and that people might totally reject the idea of reducing fat (see Chapter 4). It was, therefore, a political, not a scientific guideline. They were wrong. In my opinion, most individuals considered the guidelines to be so moderate they weren't taken seriously. This may explain why, in the years following the 1988 guidelines, only half the nation's adults and very few children had their cholesterol levels checked.

Coronary heart disease starts during childhood, and its prevention must likewise start at that time. As has already been mentioned, there can be no doubt about this, since several landmark studies conducted in the United States (described in Chapter 18) show the appearance of fatty deposits, usually referred to as "atherosclerotic lesions," in the aorta and coronary arteries as early as age 3 among children who consume high-fat diets and have elevated blood cholesterol levels. By the early teens, these deposits are far more common, depending on the youngsters' eating habits and their cholesterol levels. Fortunately, reducing children's dietary fat reduces their cholesterol levels within a few weeks. In my own clinic in southwestern Louisiana, I consistently see significant drops in children's cholesterol levels within the first 3 months after reducing dietary fat.

The NIH and the American Academy of Pediatrics (AAP) had not yet addressed this risk of excessive dietary fat in children at the time of the First National Cholesterol Conference. The AHA, to their credit, have recommended since 1984 a diet for children in which the number of calories does not exceed 30 percent from fat and 10 percent from saturated fat. The AHA was also the first to recommend this same diet for adults, during the early 1960s. But, as you will see in the following chapters, even this is too much fat for either adults or children.

Nearly four more years passed before the NIH's NCEP made *any* statement about children's dietary fat. Finally, in 1991, the agency issued a statement that children over the age of 2 should also not consume more than 30 percent of their calories from fat. This, again, was based on what they thought parents and pediatricians would accept, completely ignoring the scientific evidence that larger reductions were necessary to prevent heart disease. The AAP issued identical guidelines in 1992. Unfortunately, this was too little and too late. During the prior two years, six separate studies had already shown that this degree of fat reduction does not significantly reduce cholesterol levels or prevent coronary-artery deposits of cholesterol.

In 1992, the Centers for Disease Control and Prevention (CDC) issued a statement that the standard adult treatment or prevention approach of the NCEP had not been effective. Only one-third of persons who needed treatment for high blood cholesterol, they said, were being identified and treated. Presumably, the "token" reductions in fat recommended by the guidelines had failed to impress the public. Furthermore, many were reading in the newspapers that saturated fat wasn't so bad after all (see Chapter 20). Misinformed, they became easy prey for the beef and dairy industries, who understandably had a strong interest in what was going on.

Due to powerful lobbying by the Beef Industry Council and the National Dairy Council, both in Washington and on the local level, practically every adult, including parents, educators, lawyers, judges, physicians, and even dietitians, has been indoctrinated since childhood in the *healthful benefits of milk, cheese, and red meat.*

For example, during the early 1960s, when several enlightened scientists suggested that milk and other dairy products were high in saturated fat and therefore promoted coronary-artery disease when consumed throughout childhood, the National Dairy Council quickly responded with all their resources and influence. President Kennedy himself made a strong statement on TV to the American people about the value of whole milk and other dairy products for the health of children and adults. Now, after another 30 years, a new generation of scientists is beginning to speak out while the National Dairy Council is again poised to strike.

After the 1988 Washington, D.C., conference, I was no longer content to stand by and watch as these inadequate guidelines were being recommended to the public. My first step was to broaden my understanding of this relationship of dietary fat, cholesterol, and heart disease still further. I visited nutritional centers and lipid (cholesterol) clinics at Harvard University, New York University, the NIH, Cornell University, George Washington University, Tufts University, and Baylor University. I was among the first 300 physicians in the nation to attend a training course on diet, cholesterol, and coronary heart disease designed and conducted by the AHA. Here I was given materials and slides to use in my own presentations with parents and physicians. Along with this excellent background material I developed my own seminar, in which I discuss the necessity of an even lower fat consumption for both children and adults. I was more certain than ever that fat must be reduced to 10–15 percent of calories, for children and adults.

At a typical seminar, I suggest that children's diets go through 4 transitional stages, each lasting 3–12 weeks, before finally reaching a plant-based diet of vegetables, fruit, legumes, and grains, with little or no animal products. These stages, explained fully in Chapter 13, gradually reduce the dietary fat to 10–15 percent of calories in the fourth stage. Saturated fat becomes negligible on such a diet and does not need to be counted. Consuming 20 percent of calories from fat would be low enough for the prevention of heart disease and fat-sensitive cancers, but at this level children's "fat taste" remains, ironically making their low-fat diet more difficult to maintain.

Beginning such a diet is infinitely easier if approached during early childhood, before fatty deposits have appeared in the coronary arteries, and before a lifelong "fat habit" is established. Children are not born with a taste for animal fat. It is *learned* early in life; whereas a "low-fat habit," firmly established by the age of 8, usually lasts a lifetime. In Chapter 13, I will give you suggestions on how to implement each stage.

With these principles you will be empowered literally to *immunize* your child against the nation's number-one killer, lengthening both her life span and health span. Despite certain myths, which I will dispel in Part One, such a diet is absolutely safe for all children over the age of 2. With adequate nonfat calories, there is no risk of malnutrition or deficiencies in calcium, minerals, or vitamins. After age 2, saturated fat and cholesterol are *not* essential nutrients. For centuries, children have thrived on such a diet in many parts of the world where coronary-artery disease has been practically unknown. In this country, vegetarian Seventh-Day Adventist children outlive the average American by seven years.

You Make The Rules!

Suppose tomorrow morning you read these headlines in your newspaper:

AMERICAN CHILDREN HAVE SHORTENED LIFE SPANS!
SCIENTIFIC BREAKTHROUGHS IGNORED BY "EXPERTS."
PARENTS DEMAND THE TRUTH!

Would you read on? The headlines are fictional, but the facts are real. While your children are growing up, awaiting them are maladies named by Dr. T. Colin Campbell, nutritional biochemist at Cornell and director of the famous China Health Study, "diseases of nutritional extravagance." These consist of heart disease, cancer, stroke, hypertension, obesity, and diabetes. Statistics show that 1 out of 2 children born today will develop heart disease, and 1 out of 3 will get cancer. Health professionals have had the knowledge to prevent this for more than 3 decades, since the AHA first brought the risk of dietary fat to their attention. As a parent, you have heard this before and suspected which foods your children should eat and which they should avoid. Yet, confident that federal health agencies will tell you the truth, you have understandably done little thus far to change their diets. Dr. Campbell, basing his conclusions on his China Health Study, described in Chapter 18, has urged parents to reduce dietary fat during early childhood before these diseases secure a foothold.

D iseases of poverty:
infectious diseases, malnutrition, and gastroenteritis

Diseases of nutritional extravagance:
coronary heart disease, cancer, stroke, hypertension,
adult-onset diabetes, and obesity

Both federal and private health agencies have access to this growing body of scientific data showing the early-childhood beginnings of these diseases, but, like all great bureaucracies, they are resistant to change. Some federal programs actually seem to be adding to the problem, by promoting even higher-fat diets than ever before. The dairy and beef industries receive several billion federal dollars each year for purchases of *surplus* food. The price paid to the beef and dairy farmers depends upon *how much fat the food contains.* Thus, the industry produces as much of the high-fat products as possible. This surplus of fat-laden beef, butter, and cheese is then given to our nation's school lunch programs, where, in accordance with requirements established by the United States Department of Agriculture (USDA), it is a part of your child's daily diet. I'm certain that this program persists because of intense lobbying by the beef and dairy industries—not the USDA's concern about undernutrition and growth retardation of American children. The *real* danger, the high fat content of these foods, fortunately attracted the attention of members of the Senate Agriculture Committee in 1994 (Chapter 17). This hopefully will lead to lower-fat USDA requirements for individual schools.

This concern that a plant-based diet may retard the growth of children has finally been refuted by ongoing nutritional studies but continues to influence strongly our nation's *official* policy. Furthermore, the beef and dairy industries are attempting to discredit the new scientific data, just as the tobacco industry did 40 years ago, when the smoking–lung-disease relationship was firmly established. There can be little doubt that these powerful industries have influenced our national health policies.

The federal government, through the NIH and private associations—chiefly the AHA and the AAP—strongly influences the nutritional decisions of your physicians, dietitians, and school health professionals. Their programs and recommendations are virtually identical, all having settled on the much-too-high "moderate-fat diet," in which 30 percent of the calories come from fat.

Over the years, these "official" guidelines for dietary-fat intake have been steadily revised *downward*. I have no doubt, after talking privately with many of the members of guideline committees, that further reductions will be made in these recommendations to approach what I am advocating in this book. But with the evidence of risk so great, you cannot afford to wait for this slow bureaucratic change; your child's entire lifetime of health is at stake. The *ultimate* guidelines will depend on you.

As parents, you are in a position to change radically the health of an entire generation. For the first time in history, with the virtual elimination of the preventable diseases of childhood, you now have the opportunity to design your child's future. *You must apply the knowledge you now possess to prevent diseases that your child cannot cure in later years.* You will not be alone in this endeavor; there are encouraging signs that primary-care physicians are beginning to take a serious look at the health hazards to your children caused by excessive dietary fat.

Your pediatrician or family doctor will almost certainly share your concern about your children's fat consumption. A genuine interest has appeared in several newsletters and professional journals subscribed to by pediatricians. Dr. Frank Oski, author of *The Portable Pediatrician* and editor of the standard textbook *Principles and Practice of Pediatrics* and the journals *Contemporary Pediatrics* and

Current Opinion in Pediatrics, expresses a strong concern for reducing children's fat intake, especially from milk. A newsletter for practicing pediatricians, *Pediatric Alert*, edited by Allen Mitchell, M.D., of Boston University and Fredrick Mandell, M.D., of Harvard Medical School, reported in its December 1993 issue that interest in children's dietary fat has been rekindled by reports confirming the high prevalence of early coronary-artery lesions in most teenagers. The article encouraged pediatricians to limit dietary fat in their patients, with the reassurance that a low-fat diet is not harmful.

What Better Gift?

When your children are adults, and in the prime of their lives, who's going to tell them that their clogged arteries, malignancies, and degenerating bodies could so easily have been prevented with the knowledge *you possessed* when they were young? *Why*, they may wonder, was their ruined health allowed to evolve while we all watched? *Why*, you should ask yourself now, should you accept the status quo when you know the dismal outcome? Robert Kennedy, during the days before his death, repeatedly paraphrased a quotation first made by George Bernard Shaw: "Most men look at things as they are and wonder, Why? I dream of things that never were and ask, Why not?"

On your child's behalf, before it's too late, I urge you to read carefully the material in the following chapters. I have implemented these dietary principles with excellent results during the last two decades of my private practice as a board-certified pediatrician. I've watched a generation of my patients grow up; and I've encountered no ill effects. Parents have been enthusiastic, and I usually succeed in reducing the fat consumption of the entire family. One mother asked, "What better gift could I give to my child?"

And, finally, to answer a question I'm often asked by the families I treat: yes, for more than 20 years I've eaten a very low-fat diet (10–15 percent of calories) consisting almost exclusively of vegetables, fruits, whole grains, and legumes.

It is useless for the sheep to pass resolutions in favour of vegetarianism while the wolf remains of a different opinion.

—*W. R. Inge (1860–1954)*
Dean of St. Paul's Cathedral, London

Part One

Twelve
Common Myths
*About Low-Fat Diets
for Children*

• • •

Alas, regardless of their doom,
the little victims play!
No sense have they of ills to come,
Nor care beyond to-day.
—*Thomas Gray (1716–71)*
English poet

Chapter 1

Myth One:
Controlling Cholesterol
Can Wait

> Forty million American children have abnormally
> high cholesterol levels.
> —*Suzanne Oparil, M.D.*
> *President, American Heart Association*

*F*orty years ago, as a second-year medical student, I performed my first autopsy. The 9-year-old girl with golden-blond hair and a slender athletic body had died, suddenly and unexpectedly, of meningitis. I was shaken, because, having been her "doctor" during the illness, I was now expected to do a careful and complete dissection of her vital organs. Such is the way young doctors-to-be learn medicine.

Near the end of the three-hour procedure, while dissecting her heart, I found something that astonished both my pathology professor and me. Within the left main coronary artery—a vessel that supplies blood to the heart muscle itself—I saw a bright-yellow thickening of the vessel's wall. Tests later confirmed what we suspected: it was cholesterol!

This was a rare finding in 1955, but during the last three decades fatty deposits have been found in the coronary arteries of children with increasing frequency, as early as the prekindergarten years.

High Cholesterol? In Children?

The American Heart Association estimated in 1993 that 36 percent of American children, ages 19 and under, had high blood-cholesterol levels—above 170 mg/dl (cholesterol is measured in milligrams per deciliter of blood). In my clinic in Louisiana, a state in which children consume slightly more fat than the national average (42 percent of calories), 4 out of 10 children over age 2 have abnormally high cholesterol levels.

What does this mean? After all, aren't heart attacks something that happen later in life, usually no earlier than middle age? It's true, heart attacks rarely occur during childhood, but autopsy studies have shown conclusively that children consuming a typical Western diet (most industrialized countries) have elevated cholesterol levels and, like the little girl on my autopsy table, develop fatty deposits within their coronary arteries.

Do these fatty deposits in children's heart arteries, parents ask, cause the heart attacks so common in adults? The answer is almost certainly that they do. *In every nation of the world where children have elevated cholesterol levels—especially Finland, Northern Ireland, Scotland, England, and the United States—there is also a high death rate from coronary heart disease among the adults.* Conversely, wherever children's cholesterol levels are low, there is very little risk of coronary heart disease later, as adults. It appears that children's cholesterol levels predict this disease several decades before the first symptoms are likely to appear. Moreover, you have an even earlier predictor than these elevated cholesterol levels: your child's excessive consumption of saturated fat.

Cholesterol: The Bottom Line

The high blood-cholesterol levels, found in 4 out of 10 children in my clinic, are the direct result of too much saturated fat in the diet. How do I know this? Several carefully controlled studies, which I will discuss in more detail in Chapter 18, provide the evidence.

The NIH and the AHA list a total of 10 risk factors for developing coronary heart disease, the 4 major ones being elevated cholesterol, hypertension, smoking, and (recently added in 1992) inactivity. Though I agree that smoking, hypertension, and a sedentary life-style are undesirable, it seems to me that there is *only one* major risk factor for coronary heart disease, and it appears several decades before the first symptoms: a cholesterol level above 150 mg/dl. This is less than the upper normal limit of 170 for children set by the NIH, the AHA, and the AAP. My reasons for this benchmark level will be obvious as you read on. My opinion is shared by Dr. William Roberts, a respected scientist and editor of the *American Journal of Cardiology,* where he wrote in 1989 that there is but one true risk factor in coronary-artery disease: "All the other 'risk factors' take effect when the cholesterol level is above 150."

We can't ignore the other major risk factors doctors have been taught all these years. But after watching this disease develop in both children and adults during more than four decades, spanning two generations, I have concluded that the other 9 risk factors are only *related* to coronary heart disease *when the cholesterol level remains above 150.* This statement will surely cause ground tremors under the Dallas headquarters of the AHA.

There's only one risk factor:
a cholesterol level over 150.

To illustrate the difference between a condition or an event only *related* to heart disease and a true risk factor, let's look at the effect of natural disasters and acts of war upon susceptible individuals with high cholesterol levels. According to a study by the University of Naples, Olivetti factory workers with elevated cholesterol levels had more heart attacks after earthquakes. The Israelis, during the Iraqi missile attack of January 17–25, 1991, recorded an enormous increase in heart attacks among those people who had elevated cholesterol levels. Obviously, earthquakes and missile attacks are not heart-disease risk factors for healthy people with cholesterol levels under 150. Likewise, shoveling snow is not a heart-disease risk factor, though people with elevated cholesterol levels have heart attacks during this activity.

As for smoking and hypertension, both are common among rural Japanese men—60 percent are smokers—who have very little coronary disease on their low-fat diets and cholesterol levels well under 150.

Many of my colleagues have failed to realize just how important cholesterol levels are in predicting coronary heart disease. When I tell them that they can *absolutely* prevent heart attacks by keeping their patients' cholesterol levels under 150, they don't believe me. When I go on to tell them that keeping adults' cholesterol levels under 150 is easy when a low-fat diet is started during childhood, they think I'm being simplistic.

Then I tell them about the famous Framingham Study. Dr. William Castelli, director of the study, in which heart disease has been researched among the adult citizens of Framingham, Massachusetts, for the past 45 years, told me at a scientific conference in 1991, "We've never had a heart attack in Framingham in anyone with a cholesterol level under 150." (More recently, there have been five, all with other complications, usually diabetes.)

This strong and unconditional statement is reassuring to those of us who have devoted our professional lives to teaching people that a low-fat, high-fiber diet consisting of vegetables, fruits, whole grains, and legumes—a necessity for most individuals to reduce their cholesterol level to 150 or below—is especially effective when initiated during childhood, before the fat habit is established.

During an interview by Dr. Neal Barnard, for his book *The Power of Your Plate*, Dr. Castelli said that this diet "is consumed by three-quarters of the people who live on the earth [who] never have a heart attack. They live outside the big cities and their cholesterol levels are 150 or below." Castelli said that in our own country vegetarian men outlive meat-eaters by about six years.

Dr. Castelli added later in a *McCall's* interview, "Of the 5.3 billion people in the world, 4 billion virtually never have arteriosclerosis or colon cancer. These 4 billion people have one thing in common: They eat a low- or no-meat diet that's also very low in saturated fat, about 12 to 15 grams of [total] fat a day, as opposed to the 40 or 50 grams that are eaten daily in the United States."

When the low cholesterol levels attained by this type of diet begin in childhood and are accompanied by other good life-style habits such as avoiding tobacco and alcohol, even greater longevity can be expected. Dr. Hans Diehl, of the Lifestyle Medicine Institute in Loma Linda, California, has estimated, from all studies reported, that Seventh-Day Adventists—half of whom are vegetarian from childhood and practically none of whom smoke—live seven years longer than non-Adventists. Very low cholesterol levels (under 150) are commonly found in both children and adults who are vegetarian Seventh-Day Adventists.

If cholesterol levels are controlled in children, the probability of keeping levels below 150 later in life is much greater. In people whose cholesterol levels were above 150 in childhood, the level usually increases by 50 mg/dl by the time they reach adulthood. For example, a moderately elevated childhood level of 170–180 typically reaches 220–230 in adulthood; *the average cholesterol level measured at the time of the majority of heart attacks is between 220 and 240.*

Adult Cholesterol-Risk Levels

Satisfactory   .... Below 200
Borderline risk   200–239
High risk   .... Over 240

From NIH and AHA guidelines

These are the adult cholesterol-risk levels set by the National Cholesterol Education Program (NCEP) of the NIH. It is an interesting fact that more heart attacks occur in the borderline levels than at high-risk levels, suggesting that these benchmarks are probably set too high. It follows that the borderline-high level set by the NIH and AAP for children (170–199; see below) is also too high.

What's High, What's Not?

In my clinic, where we are always talking about cholesterol levels, parents want to know, "How high is high?" Most adults have heard that a cholesterol level below 200 mg/dl is considered desirable in adults. But parents want to know, "What's high for children?"

According to the present guidelines of the Children's Treatment Panel of the NCEP, as well as the AHA and the AAP, children under age 19 should have cholesterol levels below 170 mg/dl. Borderline high has been designated as 170–199, and 200 or above is high. But these levels would be considered high in rural Japan and China; highs in these regions would compare to our lows. And the "normal" cholesterol level of a Kalahari bushman is 77 mg/dl.

Current Guidelines for Children's Cholesterol Levels

Satisfactory .... Below 170
Borderline high 170–199
High .... 200 or above

From NIH, AHA and AAP guidelines

An Ideal Cholesterol Level

In my opinion, a cholesterol level of 150 or below is desirable in both children and adults no matter where they live. At this level, coronary heart disease rarely appears—among the rural Chinese and Japanese, or among vegetarians within Western countries. And we know that no heart attacks have been found in subjects of the Framingham Study whose levels are below 150.

Controlling Children's Cholesterol Levels

Another question a prudent parent may ask: are children with high cholesterol levels going to maintain them into adulthood, and will children with normal or low cholesterol levels maintain these as adults? The Bogalusa Heart Study, which has followed children's cholesterol levels for more than 22 years (see Chapter 18, page 154), concluded that the answer to both questions is "yes."

Cholesterol Levels and Heart-Disease Risk

The NCEP concluded that, among adults, for every 1 percent cholesterol levels were reduced, the risk of developing coronary heart disease was reduced by 2 percent. Members of the NCEP committee have expressed to me personally that this percentage may be larger, up to 3-percent risk reduction. It stands to reason that even greater heart-disease reduction may be expected for children, since *preventing* coronary-artery fat deposits is much easier than *reversing* them or even *arresting* them once they have cluttered the arteries. I would venture to say that, for every 1 percent children's cholesterol levels are reduced, their risk for developing coronary heart disease as adults is reduced by at least 4 percent. This is not an unreasonable assumption.

Reducing a child's risk by 4 percent for each 1-percent reduction in his cholesterol level may have dramatic consequences for the children I find in my practice with a "high-risk" cholesterol level of 200. A 20-percent reduction, which has proved to be easily attained by following my diet recommendations, *would reduce the child's cholesterol to 160 and reduce the risk of developing coronary heart disease as an adult by 80 percent!*

> I am confident that, because of the extra leverage of prevention, for every 1 percent children's cholesterol levels are reduced, their risk for developing coronary heart disease as adults is reduced by at least 4 percent.

The Power of Prevention

This highly favorable ratio of 1:4 gives us a precious window of opportunity for prevention before the disease gains its foothold. Once coronary-artery disease is established in adults, enormous amounts of money cannot effectively cure it. The "cure" approach, however, has unfortunately become a standard throughout the industrialized, Western nations. Since 1970, bypass surgery has gone up 2,800 percent, accounting for a large portion of the enormous annual price tag of this disease. Actually, money can't buy one's freedom from a damaged heart brought on by a childhood of poor eating habits.

AHA statisticians estimate the total annual cost of heart disease alone, in the United States, to be more than $117 billion, including charges for physician, nursing, hospital, and nursing-home services and for medication, plus the estimated cost of loss of productivity. If a preventable industrial accident were costing the nation this much, it wouldn't be tolerated.

"It is a fable for our times," wrote Neville Hodgkinson in the *London Times Magazine* (October 4, 1992), "a multi-million dollar, high-tech exposition of scientific optimism, of the belief that with enough money and know-how and aggression, the seemingly malevolent side of Mother Nature's face can be made benign."

Yet most coronary heart disease, stroke, adult diabetes, hypertention, obesity, constipation, and 50 percent of all cancers are preventable at a cost—mainly for education—totaling less than 5 percent of the annual cost of treating these disorders. Like prenatal care, childhood immunization, and counseling about exercise and smoking cessation, most health-care experts agree that educational programs to reduce the fat in children's diets save far more than they cost. Dr. Steven Woolf, a science adviser to the United States Preventive Services Task Force of the Public Health Service, said at a news conference that nutritional counseling is more effective than disease screening and early-detection programs.

If our government is sincere about reducing medical cost, then its massive resources *must* be directed to reducing children's consumption of fat. Prevention of these diseases, like prevention of infectious diseases with immunizations, *must* begin early to achieve the greatest cost-effectiveness.

First, however, we must *identify* those children with elevated cholesterol levels. At present, two-thirds of Americans with high cholesterol levels never get dietary counseling, because they don't have their levels tested. If these elevated cholesterol levels are first detected during childhood, before eating habits are firmly established, the problem won't exist.

Pediatricians Must "Discover" Cholesterol

In my experience, very few pediatricians and family doctors check the cholesterol levels of their young patients. Even those who follow the present guidelines of the NIH and the AAP do not check children's cholesterol levels unless there is a family history of coronary heart disease. Often, enlightened parents must ask for the test. Otherwise, their children would not have their cholesterol levels checked during their formative years. Pediatricians, like most other practicing physicians, have become more oriented toward treatment than prevention, and this can be corrected only by education and demands from an informed public.

Parents in my clinic have shown alarm when I find elevated blood-cholesterol levels in their children. I explain that high cholesterol levels have been proved to damage the arteries of the heart by the early teenage years if not corrected. I often use the autopsy data reported from the Korean and Vietnam wars, which showed that the *majority* (70 percent) of young—average age 20 to 22— apparently healthy soldiers killed in action had coronary-artery disease. Since this disease develops over many years, the changes in their hearts *had* to have begun in childhood. Their Asian counterparts, who had eaten low-fat diets since childhood, had clean, smooth arteries. This fact strongly impressed me when I first read the reports. It also impresses the parents of my patients.

In my practice, once I find a high cholesterol level in a child, I often check the rest of the family; I usually find a high level in at least one parent. Often, dangerously elevated levels have been discovered in parents and even grandparents. It seems to me that this approach—checking *all* members of the family—is best; it helps the children and also the parents. But this is the *opposite* approach from that suggested by the NIH in 1991 and the following year by the AAP. Their "official" guidelines recommend checking cholesterol levels only in children whose parents or grandparents have had cornary heart disease or elevated cholesterol levels. I will discuss in Chapter 18 why this is absolute nonsense. By following the

AAP guidelines, the 47,000 members of that organization will over-look half of all children with high cholesterol levels.

Judging from the preface of the 1992 edition of the *Pediatric Nutrition Handbook*—prepared by the AAP's Committee on Nutri-tion for their member pediatricians—high cholesterol levels and the risk of coronary-artery disease are not a great concern of the acad-emy: "We have come to recognize that some chronic disorders of adult years such as hypertension and dental caries [cavities] have antecedents in childhood and that it may be possible to modify the development of these disorders by changes in child nutrition." Nothing is said about the relationship of high cholesterol levels to coronary heart disease, strokes, hypertension, diabetes, or cancer.

Three Generations of Heart Attacks Prevented

Let me give you an example of how the procedure of screening *every* child is superior to the official AAP and NIH recommenda-tions. As part of an annual physical examination, a routine choles-terol test was done in my office on a 3-year-old boy. His level (210 mg/dl) was confirmed by another test a month later. Subsequently, the entire family—three older children, the mother, and the father —were checked, and all were at the high-risk level; the father's level just over 300 mg/dl.

The parents, who had not been aware of cholesterol problems or heart disease among any other members of the family, were counseled along with their older children about a reduced-fat diet. Within three months, all but the father had normal levels.

I encouraged him to bring in *his* parents, who were both living and apparently well. Neither had ever had his or her cholesterol level checked. Both had levels above 240, placing them in the high-risk category as well. After another three months on the low-fat diet, the father's and both grandparents' cholesterol levels remained high. Finally, after an additional three months in which none of them responded to a low-fat diet, I placed them on a cholesterol-lowering drug, Questran, which reduced their cholesterol to normal levels after only one month. Today, the mother and children continue to do well on their low-fat diet alone, while the father and grandparents are doing well on their diet and Questran.

This example illustrates how the high cholesterol levels of children, their parents, and their grandparents can be identified, and how intervention with diet and drugs can prevent life-threatening diseases that would otherwise progress, totally unrecognized. Recent studies have confirmed that reducing the cholesterol levels of the elderly lessens their risk of coronary disease and stroke, just as it does in young and middle-aged people.

Found: High Cholesterol. Now What?

As discussed, children above the age of 2 should have a cholesterol test, at least once. I usually do it shortly after they reach their second birthday, or at whatever age they come into my practice. This test can be done in a doctor's office with a finger-stick drop of blood, a procedure which costs the doctor $2.50 or less, depending on the type of laboratory equipment he has available. It does *not* require fasting, so it can be done at the time of any routine office visit.

For all children with levels over 170, the test is repeated on the next visit. If the second test is also elevated—as it is in at least 3 out of every 10 children tested in America—a *lipid panel* should be done on another day, after the child has fasted for 12 hours. This lipid panel, which consists of cholesterol, high-density lipoprotein (HDL), and triglyceride levels, is used to calculate the *low-density lipoprotein (LDL)*. About 65 percent of the blood cholesterol exists as LDL, which is the only form of cholesterol capable of penetrating the walls of the coronary arteries. For this reason, LDL has justly earned the name "bad cholesterol." HDL, commonly called "good cholesterol," transports cholesterol from the artery walls back to the liver for excretion. Approximately 25 percent of blood cholesterol exists as HDL. Triglycerides, which are tiny fat globules, constitute the remainder of blood cholesterol, and about one-fifth of each triglyceride globule is made up of cholesterol. Therefore, the LDL is calculated by the following formula:

$$LDL = Cholesterol - (HDL + \tfrac{1}{5}\ Triglycerides)$$

Why go to all this trouble, you may ask, to get the lipid panel and then calculate the LDL? Why not just get a cholesterol level and be done with it? Though it is true that a cholesterol level alone is a very good indication of risk, the LDL is an even better one. It is possible to find a high LDL in a child with normal (under 170) cholesterol.

LDL is harmless when found in levels under 100 mg/dl. On the other hand, levels over 110 may, over time, produce coronary-artery damage. *Such levels in children are never to be ignored.* These youngsters should be placed on a low-fat diet such as the one discussed later on in this book.

The "good" cholesterol, HDL, has received a great deal of attention in recent years. Parents have been told that low levels (below 35 mg/dl) of this type of cholesterol are likely to cause heart disease. This is true *only* when the LDL is high. If the LDL is maintained at an ideal, under 100—which corresponds approximately to a total cholesterol level of 150—by a low-fat diet of vegetables, fruit, grains, and legumes, HDL is not needed and low levels are not associated with heart disease in children or adults. Therefore, *for children or adults, a low HDL isn't an indication of risk unless the cholesterol level is above 150 or the LDL level is above 100.* Low HDL levels are common among individuals with cholesterol levels under 150, such as the rural Chinese and vegetarian groups in Western nations who have a very low risk for coronary heart disease.

Once a child is put on this new low-fat diet, the LDL level should be rechecked every three months, until it falls below the high-risk benchmark of 110. Once these safe levels are reached, LDL levels should be checked once a year.

Controlling High Cholesterol Levels

Reducing the saturated-fat content of children's diets reduces their blood-cholesterol levels, a fact still not accepted as proved by some pediatricians and family physicians. Many health-care professionals have either overlooked the published scientific studies or have succumbed to the deluge of information supplied by the beef and dairy industries, which de-emphasize the effect of saturated fat on cholesterol levels in the typical diet.

The effect of reducing the saturated-fat content of typical family meals was proved first in 1972 by an excellent diet-intervention study of 484 boys attending St. Paul's School, a boarding school in Concord, New Hampshire. The students were given a reduced-saturated-fat diet throughout the school term, but ate a typical American diet at home during spring break and summer vacation. Before they entered the study, their average cholesterol level was 178, which would have been borderline high by today's AHA standards. After only 16 days at school, their average levels dropped to 150. After a two-week spring break, when most of the students were at home, their average cholesterol levels rebounded to 186. Then, 23 days after they returned to school and the low-saturated-fat diet, the average level went down to 152, where it remained until they left for summer vacation. Finally, when they returned to school in the fall, their average cholesterol levels went back up to 183. Other, more recent studies (described in Chapter 18) have confirmed these findings.

Saturated fat raises blood-cholesterol levels.
Reducing saturated fat
reduces blood-cholesterol levels.

Cholesterol in food—and it is found only in food of animal origin, such as meat and dairy products—tends to raise the blood-cholesterol level much less than does saturated fat: only about 15 percent of cholesterol in food is absorbed into the bloodstream. On the other hand, most foods high in cholesterol are also high in saturated fat, which is readily absorbed.

The high cholesterol levels found in more than one-third of American children aren't, for the most part, the result of excess cholesterol consumed in the diet. Most of the body's cholesterol is made by the liver. The liver also takes it away, by filtering it out of the bloodstream through millions of little areas on liver cells called *LDL receptors.* Saturated fat shuts down these liver LDL receptors, and the result is rising cholesterol levels in the blood.

Therefore, if *no* cholesterol were consumed, a child could still have a high blood-cholesterol level because of the saturated-fat-suppressed cholesterol (LDL) receptors in the liver. Foods advertised as containing *no* cholesterol are misleading to the consumer if they contain, instead, excess saturated fat.

In my seminars, I often point out that shrimp, though high in cholesterol, is *very* low in saturated fat. Wild game contains as much cholesterol as domestic beef, but its saturated-fat content is far less. Even eggs, very high in cholesterol, are relatively low in saturated fat and may, in moderation, not raise cholesterol levels.

On the other hand, foods prepared with coconut oil may be cholesterol-free but are extremely high in saturated fat and cause dangerous elevations of the blood-cholesterol level. These distinctions are not understood by most consumers and even some physicians.

A decrease of cholesterol in the diet of 100 mg per 1,000 calories consumed produces a decrease in the blood-cholesterol level of about 10 mg/dl. Each 1-percent decrease in calories from saturated fat in the diet produces a decrease in the blood-cholesterol level of approximately 3 mg/dl. Saturated fat is obviously the real villain.

The major sources of saturated fat in the Western diet are dairy and meat products. Certain vegetable oils—such as coconut, palm, and palm-kernel oil—also contain high levels of saturated fat, but no cholesterol.

Fat Saturation Is the Key to Cholesterol Control

The *saturation* of fat is determined by the hydrogen atoms attached to each carbon atom of the fatty-acid molecules of which the fat is composed. *Saturated* fatty acids have a hydrogen atom attached to every carbon position. Some fatty acids have carbon atoms missing hydrogen atoms in one position, and these are known as *monounsaturated* fatty acids. Others, *polyunsaturated* fatty acids, have missing hydrogen atoms in two or more carbon positions.

Hydrogenated fat is made by adding hydrogen atoms to either mono- or polyunsaturated fat, creating compounds known as *trans fatty acids*. This hydrogenation process hardens a liquid oil, making it easier for cooking and spreading, and extending its shelf life. Examples include peanut butter and margarine. As you may already have suspected, hydrogenated fats (composed of trans fatty acids) have been found to increase cholesterol levels. They should be considered as saturated fat and avoided. These trans fats may be worse than regular saturated fat, because they raise cholesterol and lower HDL. Saturated fat raises cholesterol and HDL. Dr. Walter Willett of the Harvard School of Public Health estimates that hydrogenated fat is responsible for more than 30,000 heart disease deaths per year. Just watch for the words "hydrogenated" or "partially hydrogenated" on the label.

The fat in the foods your child consumes is made up of varying amounts of saturated, monounsaturated, and polyunsaturated fatty acids. The fat very high in saturated fatty acids is usually solid at room temperature, such as that contained in meat and butter. Those highest in monounsaturated fatty acids, such as olive oil and canola oil, are liquid at room temperature. Fats high in polyunsaturated fatty acids, such as safflower, sunflower-seed, corn, and soybean oil, are also liquid at room temperature. The thing to remember is that no dietary fat is all one type; each is a mixture of all three. For example, olive oil is composed mostly of monounsaturated fatty acids but also has a significant portion (14 percent) of saturated fatty acids.

Some authorities believe that polyunsaturated and monounsaturated fats have a *direct* effect on reducing cholesterol levels. Having reviewed the published studies, I find it more likely that this cholesterol-lowering effect occurs only because the increased polyunsaturated or monounsaturated fat consumed *replaces* saturated fat in the diet; it is the reduction of saturated fat in the diet that reduces blood-cholesterol levels. Asians' and Mediterraneans' replacement of saturated fat by either of the two other fats appears to explain why these two widely diverse cultures have very little coronary heart disease. As discussed below, Italians use more olive oil, thus less saturated fat. Asians consume less of all three kinds of fat.

Similarly, it appears that many of the supposed cholesterol-lowering effects of foods and supplements such as fish oil, beta-carotene supplements, red wine, garlic, walnuts, and oat bran may be due, in part, to the simple fact that they replace some of the saturated fat normally in the diet. Dr. Thomas Pearson, a Columbia University scientist and editor of the respected journal *Annals of Internal Medicine,* wrote in an October 1993 editorial that the primary measure for controlling cholesterol is *replacing saturated fat* rather than supplementing the diet with substances that may have some direct cholesterol-lowering effect.

The Mediterranean or the Asian Way

Children in rural Japan and China usually live on a diet with less than 10 percent of their calories from fat. Even throughout middle and old age, there is very little coronary-artery disease outside the large cities, where diets have become Westernized.

Japan claims the longest life expectancy of any nation on earth. In China, children and young adults, who have survived infectious diseases, diarrhea, and accidents, have a *remaining* life expectancy exceeding that of most Western, industrialized nations. The China Health Study (see Chapter 18) revealed no ill effects when a diet of grains, fruit, and vegetables was consumed from early infancy. Furthermore, the Chinese consumed 30 percent more calories than Americans, but no obesity was found. The Chinese diet also contained three times more fiber than Americans consume, which likely explains the rarity of colon cancer among the Chinese. The freedom from heart disease and cancer and their longevity edge are lost by Chinese children when they move with their families to large cities such as Singapore or migrate to America.

The diet consumed by children of several Mediterranean countries is low in saturated fat, but not total fat. Children in Greece, Capri, Italy, southern France, and Morocco consume nearly 40 percent of their calories as fat, mostly as monounsaturated fatty acids in olive oil. Coronary heart disease is, as in Asia, rare. On the island of Crete, for example, coronary heart disease is virtually unknown, although its inhabitants' diet derives 35–40 percent of its calories from fat.

These two cultures, the Asians and the Mediterraneans, have a dietary common ground, despite their differences in total fat intake: *a very low consumption of saturated fat, and a high intake of vegetables, fruits, and grains.* The healthful effects of olive oil and other monounsaturated fats, in my opinion, have been exaggerated in recent years. These are still 100-percent fat, and therefore high in calories. The Asians seem to have the more ideal diet, with their low levels of *all* fat throughout life.

It should be obvious by now that controlling cholesterol cannot wait. Though not apparent until years later, coronary-artery disease begins during childhood and can be prevented only by reducing saturated dietary fat during these early years.

Chapter 2

Myth Two:
Controlling Obesity
Can Wait

> Obesity in childhood is of growing concern
> because its prevalence has been increasing
> over the past two decades.
> —*Dr. Ernst L. Wynder*
> *President, American Health Foundation*

"*H*ealth is three things," says Dr. Walter Bortz, a professor at Stanford University Medical School, "good nutrition, adequate rest, and ample exercise." It's that simple, insists this 64-year-old physician, teacher, writer, vegetarian, and marathon runner, though he adds a fourth ingredient: not doing anything to hurt yourself. Two of Dr. Bortz's ingredients, nutrition and exercise, are equally important in controlling excessive weight gain throughout childhood. Whereas high cholesterol levels may not be recognized without testing, obesity is usually obvious to parents and peers. It is probably the *earliest* visible sign of poor health.

After-School Habits

I usually start my counseling of the overweight child with the question "What's the first thing you do when you get home from school?" Invariably, the answer is that she looks for something to eat. I ask if she could stall the eating until supper time, since this is only two hours later. Then I ask if she could pass this time by walking, biking, skating, or simply running errands. In my experience, children are willing to give this a try. Only when this new habit is established do I talk about changing the kind of food they eat at mealtime.

The next thing most children do when they get home from school, often to an empty house, is to turn on the television. There is a direct relationship between excessive weight gain and the number of hours of daily TV watching. Dr. C. Richard Conti, author of *Heart Disease and High Cholesterol*, estimates that each additional hour spent watching TV increases the prevalence of obesity by 2 percent. This would be expected, since children watching TV are less active. According to Dr. Dorothy Singer of the Yale University Family Television Research and Consultation Center, preschoolers average 23 hours weekly in front of the TV; elementary-school students, 29 hours; and junior high and high school students, 13 hours. Obesity researcher and nutritionist Dr. Freddie Kaye of Tallahassee, Florida, estimates that a typical child watches 5 hours of TV per day, not counting the hours spent on video games and personal computers.

There's another risk for the child who spends a lot of time in front of the TV: exposure to the food commercials. The portion of TV commercials for food deriving one-third or more of their calories from fat is increasing, according to the report of pediatric cardiologist Dr. Thomas Starc. He told the 1993 annual meeting of the AHA, in Atlanta, that these "high-fat" commercials constituted 41 percent of the total commercials shown on Saturday mornings in April 1993, compared with 16 percent in 1989–90.

The "Well-Fed" Look

Parents and grandparents who bring their children to my clinic are more often concerned about *failure* to gain weight than about gaining excess weight. "Chubby" children are still, unfortunately, often considered healthier than their slender peers.

That this would be a common attitude in the last decade of the twentieth century, when the risk of obesity is so well known, I find difficult to understand. But parents and grandparents are not entirely to blame. Even many family physicians and pediatricians have not, until recently, recognized that a child's excessive weight gain is a serious enough problem for them to offer parents the proper counseling.

No one denies the evidence that overweight children are more likely to become overweight adults with increased risk of heart disease and the other chronic degenerative diseases. This predictability of excessive weight extends all the way back to early infancy. A 1976 report in the *New England Journal of Medicine* offered proof that chubby infants were more likely to become obese adults. More recently, the Bogalusa Heart Study (see page 154) found that obesity, like elevated cholesterol levels, "tracks" into adulthood.

In his classic book, *Dr. Spock's Baby and Child Care*, the author warns that obesity is a serious problem to be corrected as soon as it appears. He advises that if a baby is becoming unusually plump, even during the first year, this shouldn't be considered cute, but should be treated with dietary shifts right away. He concedes that it may be difficult if relatives and friends tend to find fat children more attractive and healthier.

8-Year-Old Gridiron Monsters

The shocking "value" of excessively overweight boys on the local "peewee" football team was brought to my attention when, ever searching for ways to create monster 8-year-olds, Little League football coaches began sending children and their parents to my office for a drug known as Periactin. This usually harmless antihistamine is used to help control itching in chicken pox or allergic skin rashes—I've considered it as an alternative to Benadryl, because it may not cause the undesirable side effect of drowsiness. However, another effect of the drug, usually known only to doctors, had been discovered by the coaches: Periactin strongly stimulates the appetite and produces a weight gain through overeating. Some Little League players were becoming "stars" after putting on an excess of 20–30 pounds.

I was stunned to learn this, and my initial assumption that it was a local, isolated practice was wrong. I was later told by Dr. Bruce Woolley, a pharmacologist at Brigham Young University, that he had encountered the practice in his capacity as consultant to sports associations. Children, he said, were actually run through poison ivy by some enterprising coaches to create a severe rash and justify prescriptions for Periactin at their physicians' offices. Dr. Woolley has also encountered the use of a human growth hormone by children to achieve greater weight and growth for athletics.

As parents, you should strongly reject this practice, considered by many Little League coaches as harmless. Obesity at any age is unhealthy. Will such attempts to "beef up" preteens lead to encouraging the use of anabolic steroids later, in high school and college? The drugs are completely different, but the intent is more or less the same.

Some coaches have also convinced parents of my patients to hold children back a year (for "academic maturity") so that the children could be that much larger than their peers before their junior-high football career. In no other sport, with the possible exception of sumo wrestling, is this unhealthy accumulation of body fat considered an asset.

Eat Now, Diet Later?

Some parents have insisted to me that their overweight children will have plenty of time to "grow out of it." They point out other family members who were fat as children but now, as adults, have lost the weight. This may be wishful thinking, in light of recent findings about excessive weight in children and adolescents. Dietary fat during childhood may be more life-threatening than was originally suspected. Excessive body fat appearing at two periods of childhood—during infancy, or later during adolescence—may increase the number of permanent fat cells. Later weight loss just shrinks them but doesn't take them away. This increased number of fat cells essentially remains in place for a lifetime, ready to absorb excess fat. So your child may not be able to eat now and diet later without a future health hazard.

A Tufts University study by Dr. Aviva Must (an epidemiologist at the university's Department of Agriculture's Human Nutrition Research Center) reported in 1992 that adolescent obesity in males is associated with a much higher death rate (*double*) from heart attacks, strokes, and colon cancer by age 70 than among their peers of normal weight, even when the youngsters later lost the excessive weight. The death rate was also higher than when obesity had its onset later when they were adults. Dr. Must insisted that obesity must be prevented during childhood, rather than trying to reverse it later on.

A child's obesity health risks remain, even if the weight is lost later in life.

The increased number of permanent fat cells created during infancy and again during adolescence is probably the chief reason for the gradual weight gain in adults as they age, reduce their physical activity, and experience a metabolic slowdown. For example, old photographs of John Kennedy, Lyndon Johnson, and Richard Nixon as congressmen contrast sharply with later, presidential photos. Although none of them became seriously obese, the change in body weight is obvious and striking.

This weight gain over the decades of adulthood is neither normal nor inevitable. When the excessive numbers of fat cells are prevented during childhood by a low-fat, high-complex-carbohydrate diet—which likely continues for a lifetime—there is little excess fat consumed, and fewer fat cells into which it may be deposited. Also, as I will discuss later, this kind of food isn't easily converted into body fat.

Childhood Obesity Is Increasing

The Tufts University study took both parents and pediatricians by surprise. Now we can no longer ignore excessive weight gain with the hope of reversing it later on. So how're we doing? According to a survey by the American Health Foundation, 25 percent of all children were overweight in 1993. There are more obese American children now than ever before (about 20 million, estimates AHA president Dr. Suzanne Oparil). The Bogalusa Heart Study reported that the average 10-year-old is now 3.5 pounds heavier than he was 15 years ago. And, as always, most obese children are found among families of obese adults.

Since childhood obesity "tracks" into adulthood, the CDC's report in 1994 that adults between the ages of 25 and 30 are 10 pounds heavier than they were seven years earlier was not unexpected. The rate of obesity among all Americans had risen by nearly one-third during the past decade.

A Family Affair

Overweight children are usually the victims of the dietary habits of the adult members of the family. These eating habits are, in fact, passed on from one generation to the next.

While staying at a hotel in New Orleans, I watched parents and their children return repeatedly to the all-you-can-eat buffet breakfast. Food choices were almost identical for all family members—this was usually eggs and bacon or sausage. During the two hours I observed over my newspaper, practically every man had the characteristic paunch and an already overweight child. I was reminded of a comment by Neil Cusiak, champion Irish marathoner, in 1974, as we jogged across a golf course in Crowley, Louisiana: "American golfers aren't good role models for their children. They all look pregnant."

If one parent is overweight, statistics reveal, there is a 40-percent chance that at least one child will be overweight. If both parents are overweight, the chances for an overweight child increase to 80 percent. There is probably some degree of genetic influence here, but life-style habits of excessive dietary fat and too little exercise are the major reasons. Eating patterns, established by the age of 8, usually persist throughout the teenage years and into adulthood. After age 8, these habits may be changed, but with more difficulty. My "4 Stages to an Ideal Diet," described in Chapter 13, gives parents a method, using transitional stages, for changing the already established diet of an older child.

The close relationship of obesity in children to the health problems experienced by their parents and grandparents—and presumably to their own future illnesses—is illustrated by a 1991 study of 1,783 children attending schools in Muscatine, Iowa. The Department of Preventive Medicine and Environmental Health of the University of Iowa studied the causes of death of the parents and grandparents of the children studied in three groups: a lean group, a heavy group, and a group selected at random. Predictably, there was a larger number of deaths from coronary-artery disease in the parents and grandparents of the heavy children, as compared with the lean and random groups. This difference was even greater among the heavy children with above-normal blood pressure.

I find this relationship between family members to be very common among my patients. Almost always, the eating patterns of the parents play an important role and must be considered when counseling older children. For example, Elizabeth, a 12-year-old girl weighing 145 pounds, was brought in by her mother for dietary counseling. Elizabeth exceeded her ideal weight by nearly 50 pounds. She was very shy and had few friends at school. She also seemed depressed, and her academic record was poor. The mother, even though she was also at least 20 percent over her ideal weight, did not feel that she needed to make dietary changes herself. The father, I learned, was an airline pilot who had recently been placed on probation because he was over the company's upper weight limit. It was obvious that their daughter's eating habits were influenced by their own.

Finally, after several visits, I convinced both parents to join Elizabeth in our counseling sessions. All three had elevated cholesterol and LDL levels. First they were given the basic information about the surplus calories produced by dietary fat, which also has a greater propensity to be stored as body fat than do carbohydrates and protein (see pages 32–34). As the family advanced through my 4 stages of progressively lower-fat food, their weights and cholesterol levels gradually declined.

Six months later, Elizabeth had lost an average of two pounds per week and had happily reached her ideal weight. Her parents, no less enthusiastic, could see that their goal was also possible. Our counseling sessions for this family are no longer necessary, because they have adopted a diet of mostly vegetables, fruits, whole grains, and legumes. They have lost the "fat taste."

This adolescent girl's weight problem could not have been solved without the total participation of her parents. Today, all three are near vegetarians. Elizabeth's schoolwork and social life have improved, the mother has applied her new energy to work for a local charity, and the father's job is no longer in jeopardy.

Cases like Elizabeth's are often considered hopeless, since many people believe that a family such as hers is locked into a destiny of obesity by their genes. This view, which I often encounter among parents and their family physicians, dictates that essentially nothing is done. My first task is to explain the enormous power of life-style changes over the child's fixed genetic influences. We are all born with some degree of genetic burden, I tell them, but to a large degree our health is in our own hands.

Life-style changes can, in almost all cases, alter the effects of a child's genetic blueprint. One must realize, however, that this may be a double-edged sword. *Either healthy or unhealthy habits may overcome the genetic base by manyfold.* A family history of adult-onset diabetes, for example, may double a child's risk for eventually developing the disease. However, when the same child has poor life-style habits resulting in obesity, the chances of becoming a diabetic increase by 50 times.

> **L**ife-style changes can alter a child's
> genetic blueprint by manyfold.

Other physicians have experienced similar results when working with obese parents and children. Dr. William Conner, author of *The New American Diet*, a book advocating a low-fat, high-complex-carbohydrate diet of vegetables, fruits, and grains for the whole family, has devoted his entire career to the study of the effects of dietary fat. Dr. Conner feels that, too often, when children are overweight, genetics is blamed. He insists that children are usually overweight as the result of eating patterns learned from their parents. Interviewed by Dr. Neal Barnard, author of *Food for Life* and *The Power of Your Plate*, he said, "If they don't change, the kids won't change. The whole family needs to change its lifestyle."

Obesity, a Modern Phenomenon

Children haven't always had the problem with obesity that they have today. The television era worsened it sharply, but some of the changes leading to excessive weight in today's children may have started long ago.

In their book, *The Paleolithic Prescription*, S. Boyd Eaton, Marjorie Shostak, and Melvin Konner say that obesity is a modern malady of the industrial age. Paleolithic hunter-gatherers seem to have been lean, they wrote. Stone Age rock-wall paintings in Australia, North Africa, Spain, and Tanzania, as well as many figurines found in Europe and western Asia—all dating from 25,000 to 15,000 years ago—depict slender children and adults.

These people ate mostly plant foods. They ate no dairy products, and meat, irregularly available, was from wild game—containing one-third the calories and one-seventh the fat of today's domestic meat. For example, today's domesticated beef, top loin, contains 9.6 grams of fat in a 3.5-ounce serving. The same-size serving of antelope contains 2.6 grams of fat; deer, 3.2 grams; elk, 1.9 grams; and moose, less than 1 gram.

With the onset of the Agricultural Revolution, 10,000 years ago, it was no longer necessary to chase food. Domesticated animals were raised and eaten by men, women, and children, who led more sedentary lives and consumed more fat. Cows became "financial stock" which produced a product called milk, and later themselves became another product called red meat that was eaten. The age of obesity had begun.

It was not until the early twentieth century that the decrease in activity and the increase in fat consumption began to reach their unhealthy levels of today. Since 1900, the pattern of food consumption in the United States has changed drastically. Consumption of wheat, fresh vegetables, and corn is down by 41, 23, and 84 percent respectively. During the same period, beef consumption increased by 44 percent, fat and oil consumption by 49 percent, poultry consumption by 344 percent, and cheese consumption by 440 percent.

Rampant Obesity: The Last Half-Century

Finally, during the last 40 years, the typical American child's diet has deteriorated in quality to the point where the largest share of calories comes from meat, dairy products, poultry, and fish. About 20 percent of total calories are provided by snacks, far more than most Europeans—French children get 7 percent of calories from snacks. During these four decades, rampant obesity has appeared in children for the first time, and they have become heavier adults with each succeeding generation.

Changes in the seating capacity of arenas, schools, and buses graphically illustrate the problem. The great renovation of Yankee Stadium 50 years after its construction in the 1920s resulted in a capacity of several thousand *fewer* fans. The American bottom had widened by 4 inches during these 50 years; therefore, the seats had to be widened from 15 to 19 inches. For many years some of the original seats were in Mickey Mantle's Restaurant and Sports Bar on Central Park South in New York City, where most of today's customers couldn't comfortably fit into them. They look more like today's children's seats.

Classroom desks manufactured during the 1940s are hardly adequate for today's grade-school children. Dr. Bobby Stringer, superintendent of the Acadia Parish School District in Louisiana, told me that many of the very large students in his district would not have comfortably fit in the school desks used 50 years ago.

Exercise and Body Fat

Whereas cholesterol levels may be reduced by a low-saturated-fat diet alone, excess body weight is not successfully controlled without regular exercise. Active children rarely become overweight.

Regular aerobic exercise raises the metabolic rate—a process known as thermogenesis—to such a degree that during the remainder of the day and night more calories are burned per minute, even during rest. Children may, therefore, burn excess calories literally while they sleep. This has been appropriately termed by Dr. Terry Shintani, internist and nutritionist at the University of Hawaii, as "the flywheel effect."

The overweight child, whose parents are waiting hopefully for slimming as he grows older, is actually a victim of neglect. His sedentary life-style must be dealt with as early in life as possible. After he has established a regular pattern of aerobic exercise—jogging, walking, cycling, and swimming are best—a minimum of three times a week, then attention should be turned to the reduction of total fat in the diet and a concurrent increase in complex carbohydrates. Contrary to what many parents have been led to believe, complex carbohydrates are not fattening. On the other hand, simple carbohydrates (sugar, contained in cookies, candy, and cakes) may be a source of concentrated calories without other nutrients, which is why they're called "empty calories."

All Calories Aren't Alike

Excess calories from fat are converted into adipose tissue (body fat) with the help of an enzyme called lipoprotein lipase, which escorts the fat into small fat cells present from birth. The more fat cells children are born with, the easier it is for them to accumulate fat later on. This is genetically determined for each child, but, as mentioned, additional fat cells may be created during infancy and again during adolescence. Dietary fat is deposited into these cells, and this generally means that, the more fat cells children have, the greater is their tendency to gain excess weight throughout their lives.

Excess carbohydrates may also be converted into body fat, but *it is metabolically more difficult.* This is a key reason why eating the same number of calories from carbohydrates as opposed to fat does not lead to the same weight gain.

There are three ways in which eating excess fat in the form of meat, oils, and dairy products leads to more stored body fat than eating an equal amount of complex carbohydrates such as vegetables, fruit, whole grains, and legumes.

First is the simple fact that fat produces 9 calories per gram, whereas carbohydrates produce only 4. When these calories are in excess, they are stored as 1 pound of fat for every 3,500 calories. Protein, like carbohydrates, supplies only 4 calories per gram. Therefore, vegetable protein is not likely to add to excessive weight gain. Animal protein, however, is usually combined with excessive amounts of fat.

Sources of Calories

Fat produces 9 calories per gram.
Protein produces 4 calories per gram.
Carbohydrates produce 4 calories per gram.

When the above caloric densities are translated into the actual food we eat, suddenly there appears an even greater difference in calories. Whole grains and many vegetables produce less than 1 calorie per gram.

Fats and oils produce 9 calories per gram.
Meats produce 5–6 calories per gram (fat and protein).
Whole grains produce about 1 calorie per gram.
Broccoli produces 0.3 calorie per gram.

The second—and chief—reason that dietary fat produces more weight gain than complex carbohydrates is the basic difference in the metabolic rate of fat calories and carbohydrate calories, which probably accounts for the strong propensity of consumed fat to end up as stored body fat, whereas carbohydrates usually do not. The conversion of dietary fat to stored fat actually consumes fewer calories than the same conversion from carbohydrates.

To be specific, the metabolic process of storing 100 excess calories from fat as body fat requires 3 calories, so that the remaining 97 calories are stored as body fat, but 100 calories from carbohydrates require 25 calories, leaving only 75 calories to be stored as body fat.

> 100 fat calories less 3 calories = 97 calories stored.
> 100 carbohydrate calories less 25 calories = 75 stored.

Thus, it is often found that children eating *more* calories (from vegetables, fruit, grains, and legumes) weigh less than children eating fewer calories (in the form of meat and dairy products). This has also been the conclusion of a 1988 Harvard report that showed that in 8 out of 10 studies people who ate more weighed less. Dr. Dean Ornish, author of the best-sellers *Dr. Dean Ornish's Program for Reversing Heart Disease* and *Eat More, Weigh Less*, has written that his patients readily lose weight on a very low-fat, high-complex-carbohydrate diet.

The $50-billion diet industry in the United States, based almost completely on reducing calories, has chosen to ignore this basic difference between fat and carbohydrate calories.

Finally, a third reason a diet high in complex carbohydrates discourages the storage of body fat is that carbohydrates raise the metabolic rate, as does exercise. Here again, at rest, even during sleep, children on a diet of vegetables, fruit, whole grains, and legumes steadily burn excess calories.

All Fat Is Stored Equally

In the last chapter, saturated fat was emphasized because of its unique ability to raise the cholesterol level of children and adults, but remember: *all* fats, whether saturated, monounsaturated, or polyunsaturated, convert with equal ease into stored body fat.

> **S**aturated, monounsaturated, and polyunsaturated fats—they're all 100-percent fat.

The Risk Remains

The only way to avoid storage of excess calories as body fat is to consume less fat or burn excess calories through exercise. A combination of both appears to be necessary for most children. Waiting to deal with this until your child is older may, as we have discussed, allow the firm establishment of an improper eating habit and the creation of an excessive number of permanent fat cells. A shortened life span may result, even when the weight is controlled later, as an adult. Don't let this opportunity to establish healthy eating habits pass you and your child by.

Chapter 3

Myth Three:
The "Fat Taste"
Is Natural and Inborn

People who like this sort of thing will find
this the sort of thing they like.
—*Abraham Lincoln*
(1809–65)

*L*ewis Carroll, the nineteenth-century British writer of children's literature, expressed a child's cavalier sentiment toward food: " 'I'm so glad I don't like asparagus,' said the small girl to a sympathetic friend. 'Because, if I do, I should have to eat it, and I can't bear it.' " Your child's tastes in foods are dependent upon expectations learned from peers and family. She likes what she eats; so taste, created by conditioning, may change.

There Are No Fat Taste Buds

*T*he 9,000 taste buds on the tongue pick up only four basic tastes: sweet, salt, sour, and bitter. The taste buds near the tip of the tongue pick up only the sweet taste. Farther back on the tongue are the salty taste buds, then the sour taste buds, and finally, at the back of the tongue, the bitter taste buds. There are no fat taste buds. So how, you ask, do we taste fat?

Fat is "tasted" three ways: a combination of senses from the other taste buds, the sense of smell, and a food's sensation of smoothness on the tongue and within the mouth and throat. Some types of "artificial fat" (such as Simplesse, sold by the Nutrasweet Co.) have attained something similar to the fat taste by breaking down the particles into tiny globules, which is sensed as smooth by the tongue and mouth. All taste, including that for fat, is altered when the sense of smell is decreased, such as with a cold or an allergy.

Learning and Unlearning the Fat Taste

Children aren't born with a taste for fat. Studies have shown that only the "sweet taste" is present at birth. The "fat taste" is established by repeated exposure and association with pleasant experiences and social events. For example, even a 3-year-old American child has learned that cake and ice cream, not broccoli and carrots, are birthday-party foods. On the other hand, parents use fatty foods to "bribe" children to eat their vegetables. This enhances the development of the fat taste. Why, do you suppose, a 6-year-old American child savors the taste of a hamburger but a child in India is repulsed by it?

Dr. Leann Birch, at the University of Illinois's Child Development Laboratory, found strong evidence that young children learn to prefer fat by associating it with rewards and social events. High-fat foods are typically served at parties and social functions, whereas children must *earn* the right to partake in certain desired activities, such as watching television or playing outside, by eating vegetables and fruits, which parents correctly consider nutritious. Dr. Birch's studies clearly show that this produces a taste for fat and an aversion to vegetables and fruit.

Dr. Birch wrote in her report, "If you let little kids eat lots of high-fat foods, they will learn to love them. But if you expose them to low-fat foods, they often get used to them and prefer them."

Similarly, in *Dr. Spock's Baby and Child Care*, the author gives the example of a parent trying to get a child to eat a vegetable, offering ice cream only when the spinach is finished, or offering candy as a reward for finishing cereal. This creates the opposite result, says Dr. Spock, from what the parent wants: the child learns to despise spinach and cereal, and to love ice cream and candy.

Parents who raise children from infancy in a meatless, dairyless environment have effectively prevented the fat taste from ever developing by the age of 8. As discussed, reducing the fat taste becomes much more difficult after this age. In *Food for Life*, his book advocating a low-fat diet of vegetables, fruits, whole grains, and legumes, Dr. Neal Barnard wrote, "Children who acquire a taste for chicken nuggets, roast beef, and french fries today are the cancer patients, heart patients, and weight-loss clinic patients of tomorrow." This does not mean, however, that an older child—a 12-year-old, say—or even an adult cannot lose the fat taste.

Taming the Fat Taste

A taste for animal fat persists when it's consumed even in moderation. From reports of parents in my practice, I've concluded that high-fat foods actually rev a child's appetite, setting them up for a binge. On the other hand, only when animal fat isn't eaten by these children for a few weeks are they likely to develop preferences for vegetables, fruit, grains, and legumes.

So, once the "fat habit" is established, it need not be permanent. There is ample evidence that reducing or avoiding fat leads to less desire for it. The Fred Hutchinson Cancer Research Center in Seattle surveyed 448 women who had participated in group sessions to reduce the fat in their diet. Fifty-six percent of them said that while on a low-fat diet they lost their taste for fat. Sixty percent said they developed physical discomfort when they ate fat after being off fatty foods for several weeks.

A decline of taste for fat while on a low-fat diet was actually measured for the first time by Richard Mattes, a researcher at the Monell Chemical Senses Center in Philadelphia. His report compared three groups of healthy adults. The first group consumed less than 20 percent of their calories from fat. These people ate lower-fat versions of foods like meat and cheese, and no fat from condiments, such as sour cream or oily salad dressings. The second group had the same, but with added low-fat condiments. The control group was placed on a typical American diet of full-fat meats, milk, and condiments.

Beginning after 8 to 12 weeks, the group deprived of the extra fat-containing condiments and exposed to fat less frequently than the control group reported a sharp reduction of "pleasantness" ratings for high-fat foods, preferring foods with less fat content than they had before the study. Furthermore, this group developed a preference for skim rather than whole milk, which did not happen in the other study group.

Mattes said that people should try to avoid lower-fat discretionary fats in condiments and snacks because they prevent the body from getting used to low-fat foods. He added that the 8-to-12-week period the taste change required was relatively constant among the people in the study group. He concluded that once people are through this period they prefer low-fat foods.

Even occasional fat consumption maintains
the fat taste.

Are There Fat-Taste Genes?

The taste for fat quickly returns whenever we eat it. Why should this be true unless we have an *innate*, inborn desire for fat? Anthropologist E. O. Smith of Emory University says that our genes, which evolved 3 million years ago, have hardly changed since the Stone Age. He speculates that we still have the fat-craving genes that enabled our Paleolithic ancestors to survive ice-age winters. However, he said, fat was hard to come by then and accounted for no more than 20 percent of their calories (estimated by studies of today's hunter-gatherers such as the !Kung San bushmen of Botswana).

Evidence for the presence of fat-craving genes is lacking in humans, but has been found in rats by Dr. Sarah Leibowitz, a Rockefeller University neuroscientist. According to Dr. Leibowitz, galanin, a brain protein, encourages fat consumption.

David York, at Louisiana State University, reported in 1993 that he had discovered another protein, called enterostatin, which causes animals to eat *less* fat. If these two proteins exist and are active in humans, the balance between the two may explain why the fat taste is so easily learned and returns so quickly when token amounts of fat are consumed. Drug companies have expressed an interest in these findings, hoping to produce a drug for controlling the fat taste.

Searching for a chemical shortcut to tame the fat taste is typical of the scientific-industrial complex. Profit-driven pharmaceutical companies could expect billion-dollar sales for such a substance if it were placed on the market. What a waste of time, talent, and money! We already know how to deal with the fat taste, and it costs nothing: reduce fat to 10–15 percent of children's diets and the fat taste disappears for life.

Based on the studies and opinions we have discussed, it appears that the fat taste is learned by conditioning and is not an inborn trait. It can be diminished or eliminated entirely within a few weeks by reducing fat in your child's diet. The "4 Stages to an Ideal Diet" described in Chapter 13 will guide you through this transition.

Chapter 4

Myth Four:
Small Reductions
in Fat Will Do

Let us not abdicate our responsibility
to organizations and government.
—*Albert Schweitzer, M.D.*
(1875–1965)

*M*oderate reductions in dietary fat, as already discussed, do not
effectively eliminate your child's fat taste. It also appears from recent studies that this will also not significantly reduce his risk of
coronary heart disease.

The amount of fat removed by trimming meat and peeling skin
from chicken and turkey is inadequate for reducing cholesterol in
the 30–40 percent of American children with abnormally high levels. Something has to be done about milk, other dairy products,
and even the leanest cuts of meat. Snacks and desserts are major
sources of invisible or "hidden" fats (see Chapter 11). Here I will
emphasize once again that reducing fat isn't necessarily healthy unless these calories are replaced by a concurrent increase in vegetables, fruits, whole grains, and legumes. Otherwise, we simply
achieve what has been called the "jelly-bean effect"—low-fat but
with fewer nutrients.

Americans have been making *token* reductions of fat in their diets in recent years, but their consumption of fruits and vegetables is also decreasing. NPD Group, a Chicago firm that tracks eating habits, found that in 1993 only 29.3 percent of meals prepared at home included vegetables, not counting potatoes. That was the lowest level since the firm began tracking consumer behavior in 1981, a year when 34.7 percent of all meals included vegetables.

Low fat plus high complex carbohydrates = an ideal diet.

Trimming the Fat Is Not Enough

Parents often return to my office with a child whose cholesterol level is still high several months after switching from trimmed beef to skinless chicken, turkey, or fish. I explain to them that the cholesterol levels will come down after further reductions of animal fat. Often this requires eliminating poultry and fish except in small amounts, as condiments. Invariably, when this is done, cholesterol levels drop within two to four weeks.

This experience has been repeated in my clinic many times. I've not seen significant reduction of cholesterol levels in families who simply switch from red meat to poultry and fish. This should be considered only a first step in the right direction.

After reading an article in *The New York Times* that questioned the effectiveness of the AHA Step I diet (30 percent of calories or less from fat and 10 percent from saturated fat) for reducing cholesterol levels and heart disease, Dr. Gabe Mirkin, a Washington, D.C., pediatrician and author of the popular book *Getting Thin*, wrote to the editor on April 29, 1993: "For more than 30 years, the American Heart Association has been preaching—without adequate supporting data—that you only have to lower your intake of fat a little bit [to reduce cholesterol]." Dr. Mirkin's message was right on target. Americans, who consume on average 36 percent of their calories from fat—and children often exceed 50 percent—cannot significantly improve their risk by reducing fat to 30 percent of their calories. Fat must be reduced to 20 percent or even lower to prevent heart disease and cancer.

Health officials in Finland, Norway, and Sweden, as far back as 1968, were the first to make recommendations that the general public in their countries reduce their calories from fat to 25 percent. They also suggested that people increase their consumption of vegetables. In Finland, the very high coronary-heart-disease death rate is decreasing, though it still remains one of the highest in the world. Guidelines as low as the Scandinavians' have never been issued by a health agency of the U.S. government.

Recommended Fat Keeps Falling

In 1977 a Select Committee on Nutrition and Human Needs was established by the U.S. Senate (the McGovern Committee). It issued "Dietary Goals for the United States," which recommended increasing whole grains, vegetables, fruits, fish, and poultry; decreasing fatty meats, whole dairy products, eggs, and high-cholesterol foods; and decreasing consumption of sugar and salt. No specific guidelines were issued concerning the upper limits of fat. As already mentioned, the American Heart Association had made similar recommendations during the early 1960s.

The first official recommendation in our own country that dietary fat be set at 30 percent of calories or less was by the National Academy of Sciences in 1982. Dr. T. Colin Campbell, one of the authors of that document, now states that "30 percent" was chosen only to appease the public. New York University's nutrition chief Dr. Marion Nestle strongly agreed when both were interviewed by *Longevity* magazine in May 1994: "It was a compromise to appeal to the American public." Thirty percent was, however, adopted by the NIH, when the NCEP printed its guidelines in 1988.

Many researchers studying the relationship of cholesterol to heart disease have recommended 20 percent as the upper limit. This is the recommendation of Dr. Ernst Wynder, president of the American Health Foundation, and Dr. Oliver Alabaster, director of the Institute for Disease Prevention at the George Washington University Medical Center.

Finally, since 1990, studies by Dr. Dean Ornish and others suggest that fat must be reduced to 10–15 percent of calories to reduce cholesterol levels significantly and prevent new coronary-artery athrosclerotic lesions. This requires almost the total elimination of all animal products except egg whites and nonfat dairy products. Unfortunately, many family physicians and pediatricians aren't willing to ask their patients to consider this, regardless of what the scientific evidence shows.

Dr. Peter Jones, assistant professor of medicine at Baylor University Medical School, specializes in cholesterol disorders and their dietary control. "Eat nothing that walks on four legs," he said to a large group of practicing physicians at a conference in 1990. After the conference, one of the doctors joked: "Next thing he'll tell us not to eat anything that tries to get away!" He was apparently speaking tongue-in-cheek, but the fact is, most practicing physicians aren't taking low-fat recommendations seriously. The majority of pediatricians aren't even thinking about it for children.

Thirty percent of calories is too much fat.

By 1991, six studies at leading medical centers had shown that, on a diet of 30 percent of calories from fat (the current official guidelines for Americans), usually containing approximately 10 percent from saturated fat, there is a *progression* of coronary heart disease. One of these studies found the same progression of lesions in the coronary arteries on a diet with 26 percent of the calories from fat. The exception appears to be found among the Italians and Greeks, who, as discussed, consume very little saturated fat.

Timid Doctors

The cowed doctor cringed as his patient told him: "You take away my fried chicken, you'll kill me!" I cringed too, sitting at a nearby table in the hospital emergency room, because I knew what was coming next.

Intimidated, the doctor suggested that his patient just eat *less* beef, remove the skin from his fried chicken, and switch to low-fat milk. Feeling that his patient would never comply with a meaningful reduction of dietary fat, he felt justified in compromising with something he expected the patient would accept. And nothing was said about the invisible fat in desserts, pastries, cookies, candy bars, and *low-fat* milk.

Timid Government Agencies

Bonnie Liebman, of the Center for Science in the Public Interest, identifies the real reason health authorities are reluctant to tell the public how *little* fat they must eat in order to avoid heart disease: "They're afraid it will scare people off." Members of the NCEP's Adult and Child Treatment Panels have admitted privately that the committee was afraid people wouldn't make *any* change if they recommended something too drastic.

I say, give the public the facts and let them decide. Quitting smoking was known to be difficult, but health authorities didn't recommend that smokers simply cut down to a level of smoking they might have found tolerable. The National Cancer Institute instead recommended *no* smoking, because this was the only possible advice based on the facts. This kind of no-nonsense approach is needed concerning dietary fat.

The NCEP Holds Firm

Dr. Scott Grundy, chairman of the Adult Treatment Panel of the NCEP, has resisted any further reductions of dietary fat in the panel's guidelines, despite pleadings from most of the scientists who have conducted the studies proving the guidelines to be inadequate.

In January 1993, 16 heart-disease experts wrote a letter to Dr. Grundy before the NCEP issued its updated guidelines, urging that the panel further reduce their recommendation for dietary fat. The letter—signed by such renowned scientists as Dr. Dean Ornish; Dr. Gerald Berenson, director of the Bogalusa Heart Study; Dr. William Haskell, professor of medicine at Stanford University; Dr. David Blankenhorn, director of atherosclerosis research at the University of Southern California; Dr. Marion Nestle, chairman of the Department of Nutrition at New York University; Dr. Ernst Schaefer, chief of the Lipid Metabolism Laboratory at Tufts University; and Dr. William Weidman, professor of pediatrics at the Mayo Medical School—urged the committee to consider reducing *saturated* fat down to levels as low as 3 percent of calories.

The letter insisted: "Your panel could provide the leadership to let the public know about the emerging consensus concerning saturated fat. We encourage you to take this opportunity to move Americans closer to diets that would offer the greatest protection against heart disease."

The panel remained convinced, however, that any further reductions, however healthful, would be discouraging. Like Lt. Col. Nathan Jessep in the climactic courtroom scene of *A Few Good Men,* the panel seemed to be telling the public, "You can't handle the truth!"

Give Consumers a Chance

A 1992 study by Neal Barnard and Dean Ornish, published in the *Journal of Cardiopulmonary Rehabilitation,* showed that there is little difference in the difficulty experienced in reducing fat to 30 percent or to 10 percent of calories. When eating only 10 percent of calories from fat, the patients had the pleasure of knowing that they were actually preventing or even reversing coronary heart disease. Those who reduced their fat calories to 30 percent experienced progression of their disease, while having just as much difficulty adjusting to the diet.

Dr. Ornish, therefore, strongly disagreeing with the NCEP panel's reasoning, wrote in the same article, "Moderate changes give patients the worst of both worlds. They feel diet-deprived, but they don't get the positive biological changes, so they feel disappointed." He meant the kinds of changes that they could measure or perceive, such as cholesterol levels, weight loss, and feeling well.

A Stronger Voice

Whereas the NCEP's panel is afraid to make recommendations for greater reductions in fat, the Food and Nutrition Board of the National Academy of Sciences showed more courage by making an independent recommendation in 1992. In their *Diet and Health Report,* referring to NCEP's recommendations, they wrote, "The scientific evidence suggests that adults may achieve additional health benefits by cutting even more fat, saturated fatty acids, and cholesterol from their diets." They didn't comment on the NCEP's recommendation for children. But this shows that a federal agency can change its mind and say so.

Judging from the scientists who have been outspoken, such as Drs. Campbell, Ornish, Wynder, and Alabaster, the pressure is mounting, but so far the NCEP, like the cowed private doctor, is afraid that people can't handle the truth. They are underestimating the reasoning power of the general public.

These fears of discouraging the public would no longer be a consideration if low-fat eating were phased in during early childhood. Since eating properly may be easily learned only once, that's where the biggest return for our time and money can be found. Parents who never give a second thought to their own cholesterol levels are suddenly intensely interested when I tell them that their child's cholesterol is high. I've been very successful in reducing saturated fat in the diets of my young patients by simply explaining it *one time* to their parents.

Fat Should Be Taxed

I suggest that food containing excessive fat be taxed like cigarettes and alcohol. For example, any food with a per-serving fat content exceeding 4 grams would fall under the "high-fat tax." Admit it; it's a good idea. Not *all* fat, just excess fat. I say this because health statistics clearly show that excessive dietary fat causes more deaths and costs more in health care than tobacco, alcohol, and illegal drugs combined. A study from Brandeis University revealed that 500,000 Americans died from all forms of substance abuse, at a total economic cost of $238 billion in 1990. The death toll and cost from chronic degenerative diseases related to excessive dietary fat far exceeded this.

Total dollar costs and deaths from excess dietary fat far exceed costs and deaths from all forms of substance abuse, including tobacco, alcohol, and illegal drugs combined.

Taxing excessive fat in food would, in the beginning, create a windfall of vast new tax revenues, which could be earmarked for nutritional education for schoolchildren and school food-service personnel. Tax revenue would decrease slowly as less fat was consumed. For example, there has been a .25-percent drop in smoking for every 1-percent increase in federal and state cigarette taxes. But then would come the real payoff of such a plan: as fat consumption decreased, the incidence of heart disease, cancer, and other chronic degenerative diseases would drop sharply, saving hundreds of billions of dollars now spent on health care. Work productivity would increase because of less illness and absenteeism. Seven of the top 10 causes of death in America would sharply decrease, and the average life span would greatly increase.

In summary, the small reductions in dietary fat (such as those recommended by the NCEP for American children and adults) are not enough to reduce cholesterol levels significantly and prevent coronary-artery disease. Larger reductions, insists the NCEP, will discourage the public. You should be told the truth and allowed to decide for yourself. Otherwise, this apparent "Catch-22" will seal the fate of your child's health, along with that of yet another generation.

Chapter 5

Myth Five:
Children's Diets
Are Getting Better

School-age children eat the typical U.S. adult diet
characterized by high intakes of sodium, refined
carbohydrates, animal protein, and fat, and low
intakes of potassium, complex carbohydrates,
and vegetable protein and fat.

—*Dr. Gerald Berenson*
Director, Bogalusa Heart Study 1989

*I*n 1984, everyone was trying to eat less fat. The first of the large
clinical studies relating dietary fat, cholesterol, and heart disease
had been reported, and Americans were demanding lower-fat food
for themselves and their children. *Time* magazine featured on its
cover a sad face composed of a fried egg and a piece of bacon.

The Race for Children's Taste Buds

One has to look no further than the fast-food industry to see
changes reflecting consumer demand. The typical American teenager's diet practically *mirrors* that offered by the fast-food restau-

rants—up to 60 percent of calories from fat. When the food preferences of children and teenagers change, the food offered by fast-food outlets changes. Fast!

For example, by 1984, the fast-food industry, following the public demand, had introduced salad bars, baked potatoes, and low-fat burgers. McDonald's McLean Deluxe would surely soon outsell its popular Big Mac, the restaurant predicted, as it prepared for the coming "low-fat revolution." McDonald's also switched to vegetable oil instead of lard for frying. This in itself was a milestone.

Other fast-food outlets quickly brought out their own low-fat selections. Pizza restaurants, not to be outdone in this new race for children's and teenagers' taste buds, tried thinner crusts, all-vegetable toppings, and skim-milk cheese. Kentucky Fried Chicken quickly removed the word "Fried" from their logo. Now known as KFC, they promoted their Skinless Crispy, which was sold in two-thirds of their 5,089 restaurants.

These were exciting times, because fast-food restaurants had always been a major source of children's and adolescents' dietary fat. Those of us strongly advocating even further reductions in children's consumption of fat were encouraged. If fast-food restaurants were making a strong effort to reduce fat, we reasoned, surely other restaurants and even school lunch programs would follow. We were wrong.

The Fat Habit Returns

The encouraging trend was short-lived. During the late 1980s, there appeared in the media a series of reports that maybe fat and cholesterol weren't so bad after all. These ideas were the result of several poorly designed scientific studies and other well-meaning scientific reports that were misunderstood by the media, all of which will be discussed in greater detail in Chapter 20.

Predictably, the misinformed consumers—adults and their children—started buying higher-fat foods again. As a result, the low-fat food wasn't selling, so the restaurants switched back to sandwiches, burgers, and other fast food containing more beef, cheese, and fat-laden condiments than ever before. By 1989, according to an American Health Foundation monograph, the average American child's diet derived 42 percent of its calories from fat.

A Fat Rampage

Marketing experts, according to a *Wall Street Journal* article in 1993, said that Americans want *more* fat: "They are tired of the stern warning issued during the past few years by physicians and dietitians." Barry Gibbons, CEO of Burger King Corp., agreed: "Consumers have had their fill of healthier fare. They're back to Whoppers and fries." His restaurants began featuring meat loaf and fried pork.

The momentum of the low-fat trend had been broken, and America's youth went on a fat rampage. McDonald's McLean Deluxe fell to 2 percent of 1993 sales and was completely phased out in most restaurants, replaced by the giant Mega Mac, containing more beef, cheese, and fat than the 30-year favorite, Big Mac. According to the *Wall Street Journal* article, this giant contained a full half-pound of beef and was touted as "the biggest, fattest burger ever to come off a McDonald's grill." The report went on to say that "many people seem to be putting food taste before good nutrition, and that means f-a-t."

Hardee's, after watching the McDonald's experience, dropped their plans to introduce a "lean" burger. And the California-based Carl's Jr. tested a lower-fat ground-beef sandwich for several months and found little demand among their customers.

Wendy's—whose lean burger had never made it past the taste testers—hadn't taken the low-fat trend as seriously as its competitors had in the first place. They explained the new trend to a *Time* reporter: "Fat is needed to make a burger taste good." Kentucky Fried Chicken went back to Extra Crispy. Sales of *all* fried chicken consumed anywhere outside the home grew an average of 3.5 percent annually after 1989.

In 1992, retailers sold double the amount of cheese sold in 1964, and bacon sales were up another 4 percent from the previous year, to an all-time high. The dairy industry began finding new ways to increase children's consumption of whole milk (see Chapter 7) by adding flavors. Piccadilly Cafeterias, a national chain, put more bacon into its vegetables to enhance taste and demand, according to one of their managers. Egg sales were up again, following several media articles reporting studies that the cholesterol in eggs isn't as high as older tests had indicated (220 mg vs. 270 mg).

The Presidential Burger

Edward Rensi, McDonald's U.S. president, said at a nutrition conference that his company was having a great deal of difficulty communicating nutrition to customers. He thought the public's habits had changed. Meanwhile, McDonald's executives were ecstatic when the President of the United States dropped in to one of their restaurants while jogging. Newspapers had reported that the Mega Burger, first tested in the Washington, D.C., area, better suited President Clinton's "fill-me-up" appetite. Encouraged by its acceptance in the D.C. area, McDonald's made plans to offer other extra-big burgers, including the "Mickey D," containing two times as much beef as its popular Big Mac. Back at the White House, according to *The Washington Post*, Hillary Clinton has orderd veggie burgers by the case. More than 3,800 burgers were consumed in just over two months.

High-Fat Snacks Rebound

High-fat snacks continued to be big sellers at supermarkets. *Snack Food* magazine reported in 1988 that, of the $25 billion spent on snack food, $7.4 billion was for candy, $5.6 billion for cookies and crackers, $3 billion for potato chips, $1.5 billion for corn and tortilla chips, and $1.24 billion for packaged cakes and pies. Healthful low-fat snacks didn't even make the list.

So how can young consumers resist? They have been told by the media that low cholesterol levels are dangerous, that reducing fat can add only months to their life span, and that eliminating heart disease entirely prolongs life by only three years. Later on in the book, I will discuss these ridiculous reports and offer advice to bolster your children's resistance to the plethora of high-fat foods and snacks.

Chapter 6

Myth Six:
Meat Is Needed for Protein and Iron

A steak is every bit as deadly as a gun. Worse. At least if one points a gun at one's head and pulls the trigger, the end comes with merciful swiftness, but a steak—ah, the exquisite and unremitting agonies of the flesh eater, his colon clogged with its putrefactive load, the blood settling in his gut, the carnivore's rage building in his brittle heart—a steak kills day by day, minute by minute, through the martyrdom of a lifetime.

> —*Dr. John Harvey Kellogg,*
> *speaking to a group of his patients*
> *in the novel* The Road to Wellville
> *by T. Coraghessan Boyle*

*D*uring the mid-1980s, a rumor that McDonald's restaurants added earthworms to its hamburger meat was sweeping across the nation. The reason for this additive, according to this inaccurate rumor: to increase the protein content of its hamburgers. That such an unlikely idea should capture people's imagination illustrates how consumers, encouraged by the beef industries, have presumed that animal protein is needed in ever greater quantities for optimal health.

Children and adults in America obtain two-thirds of their protein from animal sources, chiefly meat. Of the one-third of protein from plant foods, about 17 percent comes from beans and grains. There is scientific evidence that this much animal protein may place our children's health in jeopardy, increasing sharply their risk of heart disease and cancer, whereas vegetable protein carries no such risk. Rural Chinese, among whom heart disease and cancer are rare, consume only 10.8 percent of their protein from animal sources.

The Animal-Protein Risk

The meat-protein risk is separate from the risk of consuming the abundance of fat contained in meat. This was essentially proved by two European studies which compared the effects of animal and vegetable protein on blood-cholesterol levels. As reported in the British journal *Lancet* in 1977, in one study animal protein was replaced with soybean protein in the already low-fat diets (which remained unchanged) of 20 people. There was a 14-percent drop in their cholesterol levels after two weeks, and by three weeks this decrease in cholesterol had reached 21 percent. These results were confirmed by another European study, in 1980, in which the same protocol was followed on 127 people, with similar results. Though their low-fat diets remained constant during the study, 67 men and 60 women had their animal protein replaced with soybean protein. After eight weeks, the males had a 23.1-percent drop in their cholesterol levels and the females recorded a 25.3-percent decrease. It appears, therefore, that animal protein has a definite cholesterol-raising effect. Furthermore, these findings are consistent with epidemiological studies, which show that populations eating more animal protein—but not more fat—have higher rates of heart disease.

Besides raising cholesterol and causing heart disease, animal protein seems to increase the risk for several cancers, especially cancer of the colon, prostate, and, breast. The National Academy of Sciences reported in 1982, in their widely respected publication, *Diet, Nutrition, and Cancer*, that animal protein "may be associated with an increased risk of cancers at certain sites." At that time, there were few studies to offer further proof. More were to come.

Dr. Walter Willett, chief of nutrition at Harvard University, after studying 88,751 women, reported that women who ate red meat every day were 2½ times as likely to have had colon cancer than women who ate meat sparingly or not at all. He concluded in a *New York Times* interview: "If you step back and look at the data, the optimum amount of red meat you eat should be zero."

Dr. Willett further commented about other meat sources of animal protein: interviewed by *Health* magazine, he said that many families, while changing their eating habits and reducing fat, have unfortunately simply changed from beef to lower-fat animal foods instead of replacing the fattier animal foods, such as beef, with grains, beans, vegetables, and fruit. Thus, eating more chicken, turkey, and fish has, while reducing fat, increased animal protein consumption, which was already too high in their diets.

Meat Outsells Vegetables and Fruit

Despite the well-publicized heart-disease and cancer risk of consuming meat regularly, marketing reports show that it still outsells vegetables and fruit three to one. Meat, in fact, leads all other foods in supermarket sales. A spokesman for the Great Atlantic & Pacific Tea Co., operators of A&P supermarkets, reports that meat generates 20 percent of their entire store sales. Combined sales of all fresh fruits and vegetables contributed only 7 percent.

Because I have tried, in my seminars and my medical practice, to puncture consumers' myths about meat, I've been accused by some people of unfairly bashing red meat. After all, the Beef Industry Council insists, even though high in saturated fat, well-trimmed servings are good for one's health. The reason given—no one can doubt the danger of saturated fat—is their *very high protein and iron content*. We have discussed the relationship of animal protein to both heart disease and cancer. Now, according to a study in Finland, iron may be red meat's most dangerous ingredient. In this study, high iron levels were found to be a major risk factor for coronary-artery disease.

The results of this five-year study, published in September 1992 in *Circulation,* the American Heart Association's most prestigious journal, found convincing evidence that iron helps LDL form the plaque in the coronary arteries by a process known as oxidation, which enables it to attach to the vessel wall more easily. According to the study, LDL that remains unoxidized may be harmless. Among 1,900 healthy men, the iron level was the second-largest risk factor, behind cigarette smoking, in those who developed coronary disease. If this is confirmed in other studies, meat may contain three lethal ingredients: fat, animal protein, and iron. However, several other studies have failed to confirm the iron–heart disease connection.

"Complete" Proteins?

Until recently, animal proteins from meat and dairy products were thought to be necessary in order to obtain what nutritionists called "complete proteins."

Proteins are composed of animo acids, 12 of which are manufactured by the human body. Another 9, called *essential amino acids,* must be obtained from food. Most animal products, such as meat and dairy products, contain *all* of the essential amino acids and have been designated as containing *complete proteins.* Most proteins from vegetables also contain all 9 essential amino acids, but 1 or 2 may be low in a particular food compared with a protein from most animal sources. Beans, however, are rich sources of all essential amino acids.

The old ideas about the necessity of carefully *combining* vegetables at every meal to ensure the supply of essential amino acids has been totally refuted. Modern nutritionists, after observing populations of strict vegetarians who were healthier and lived longer than meat-eaters, now realize that all essential amino acids may be obtained from a variety of vegetables or grains eaten over a one-to-two-day period. This should be a great relief to you as a parent. Even the variety is not as critical as once thought. Dr. Reed Mangels, nutrition editor of *Vegetarian Journal,* illustrates this by pointing out that if you decided to eat *only* six to eight potatoes you would get all the essential amino acids you would need in a single day. Of course, her example was intended only to show that combining foods daily is not critical for obtaining essential amino acids; eating only potatoes is not recommended, because a more varied diet assures you of other necessary nutrients.

> **M**eat is not necessary to ensure a supply of complete proteins.

Less than 70 years ago, more than 40 percent of the protein in the American diet came from grains, bread, and cereal. Currently, only 17 percent comes from these sources, along with another 15 percent from legumes, fruits, and vegetables, while two-thirds is from animal products. This trend, also noted in other industrialized Western countries, has been accompanied by a steady increase in heart-disease and cancer deaths.

Along with this shift to animal sources, the total protein in the diet has become excessive. The average American child's diet contains excessive protein, far exceeding the Recommended Dietary Allowances (RDAs) established by the National Research Council. A 4-year-old needs about 33 grams per day; a 12-year-old, 45 grams; and an adult, 50–65 grams. Children actually consume 50–60 grams and adults up to 100 grams, mostly from meat and dairy products. The rural Chinese adult diet consists of an ideal 55–60 grams, mostly from plant sources.

Animal Protein Is Accompanied by Fat

Children and adults need protein in amounts similar to fat, about 10–15 percent of calories, but it makes no sense to get it by eating meat. *It's impossible to get protein from red meat without also getting an abundance of saturated fat.* At least 90 percent of the protein needed in our diet can be obtained from vegetables and legumes with essentially no fat; the remainder is easily obtained from grains and fruits. For example, 2 ounces of lean ground beef supplies 14 grams of protein, but includes 20 grams of fat. On the other hand, a cup of kidney beans supplies 16 grams of protein with only 1 gram of fat. Furthermore, the ground-beef serving contains 4 grams of artery-clogging saturated fat, whereas the beans contain none. A similar amount of protein is contained in 1 cup of black-eyed peas, or of lentils, or of navy or lima beans, or of split peas, of brown rice, or 4 ounces of whole-wheat pasta. A serving of black or pinto beans contain *three times* this amount of protein. All are practically fat-free.

The lean beef, like all other animal products, contains no fiber, but the legumes listed above are rich in cholesterol-lowering soluble fiber and colon-cancer-preventing insoluble fiber. It's no wonder the American Heart Association and the American Cancer Society have given beans their seal of approval.

Vegetables Supply Plenty of Protein

In addition to the rich sources of protein from grains and legumes, already discussed above, vegetables are not far behind. Spinach, broccoli, turnip greens, collards, and kale derive nearly half of their calories from protein; and protein accounts for one-third of the calories of mushrooms, parsley, lettuce, and green peas. In fact, *all* vegetables add significant protein to the diet, leaving *none* necessary from meat and dairy products.

Cruel Joke

In all Western nations, beef has attained an unprecedented status among consumers. This has been interrupted only briefly, during the mid-1980s, when the evils of saturated fat were, for a few years, taken seriously by most knowledgeable people.

In *Beyond Beef,* Jeremy Rifkin writes: "Americans and Europeans are literally eating themselves to death, gorging on marbled beef and other grain-fed animal products, taking into their bodies massive amounts of saturated fats and cholesterol. The fatty substances are building up in the bloodstream, clogging arteries, lining cell walls, blocking passages, triggering metabolic and hormonal changes, stimulating cell growth, and rupturing organs. The 'good life' promised by the beef culture has metamorphosed into a cruel joke as Americans, overweight and plagued by the diseases of affluence, suffer from their own excesses."

The nutritional myth that meat is needed for your child as a source of protein and iron is no longer valid for the reasons discussed previously. The fact is, the ideal diet for children contains little or no meat. Animal protein, like fat, is a nutrient most children already consume far too much of, if they are on a typical American diet. Iron, like animal protein, is also likely to be excessive for children who consume meat regularly. For more than 32 years, I have been encouraging parents to reduce or eliminate their children's meat consumption. Children who don't eat meat will be, in my opinion, among those adults in the next generation with no heart disease and cancer.

Chapter 7

Myth Seven:
Milk Is Needed for Calcium and Protein

> Truth, sir, is a cow, which will yield
> skeptics no more milk; so they have gone
> to milk the bull.
> —*Dr. Samuel Johnson (1709–84)*
> *English author*

*T*he dairy industry, with all its powerful resources, has increased its spending on lobbying efforts to prove the health value of milk and other dairy products. Ironically, this renewed effort is partially due to the large body of accumulating scientific evidence indicating that just the opposite is true.

The most effective propaganda tool of the National Dairy Council is the misleading, long-standing notion that milk is a necessary source of calcium. Yet, according to Dr. Frank Oski, author of the popular textbook for doctors *The Portable Pediatrician*, milk is not a desirable part of a healthy child's diet.

The council is doing its job well, unfortunately, according to marketing data. The Food Marketing Institute reported in 1991 that 31 percent of American supermarket shoppers said they were eating less meat, and 28 percent said they were eating fewer fats and oils.

However, only 7 percent said they were eating fewer dairy products and less whole milk! *The University of California at Berkeley Newsletter* reported in January 1993 that Americans eat more than twice as much cheese today as in the late 1960s—28 pounds per person each year.

People cutting back on fat find cheese the most difficult food to forgo, according to the Berkeley report. The fat habit is nowhere more evident than in children's fondness for cheese—on such foods as pizza, enchiladas, and cheeseburgers.

Milk Can Spoil a Perfect Diet

Reducing dietary fat to levels necessary to the control of cholesterol cannot be achieved if a child drinks whole milk or eats cheese. Since these foods are major sources of saturated fat, even non–meat-eaters consuming them may have high cholesterol levels. Repeatedly, I've had children return with cholesterol levels still elevated, only to find that, after becoming "near vegetarians," they were still getting excessive saturated fat from whole milk, cheese, and various other dairy products.

Milk's Other Health Hazards

The cow's-milk protein is also one of the main causes of severe allergy, such as asthma and eczema. Furthermore, new evidence shows that it may be responsible for other serious diseases. A study by Dr. Hans-Michael Dosch, published in the *New England Journal of Medicine* in August 1992, showed that allergy to milk protein in susceptible individuals may be one of the causes of Type I (insulin dependent) diabetes in children. This is not an entirely new idea; other scientists have noted and reported, since 1990, that more diabetes is found in countries where people consume the most milk.

No other animal (except the human species) ingests milk after weaning, which suggests that milk isn't needed for developing strong bones. Animals don't get osteoporosis, but most milk-drinking girls and women develop this malady by the age of 60.

I have often removed dairy products from children's diets for a variety of reasons, chiefly to avoid allergies and to reduce saturated fat. For nearly 20 years, I have also been an advocate of reducing all fat from any source, including milk. Many of the children I have worked with are now healthy adults, and none, to my knowledge, have lacked adequate calcium and protein for healthy growth and development.

Good Intentions, but . . .

It is commonly thought, even among some dietitians, that dairy products will prevent deficiencies of the essential fatty acid linoleic acid, a necessary ingredient for cell-wall and hormone production. Actually, it's needed in only very small amounts, and is usually obtained from vegetable oils. Meat and dairy products contain very little. Furthermore, according to an article in the *Journal of Pediatric Gastroenterology,* cow's milk does not meet the nutritional needs of a child under 1 year of age. It's deficient in some nutrients and contains too much of others.

Most pediatricians have continued to recommend cow's milk for their infant patients beginning from 6 months to 1 year. This may soon change, since the usually pro-milk AAP's Committee on Nutrition issued a statement to its member pediatricians in June 1992 concerning children under the age of 2:

> *Infants fed whole cow's milk have low intakes of iron, linoleic acid, and vitamin E, and excessive intakes of sodium, potassium, and protein, illustrating the poor nutritional compatibility of solid foods and whole cow's milk.*

Whole cow's milk *displaces* some and, in many cases, most solids in this age group. I regularly find children in my practice over the age of 1 year who consume up to a half-gallon of cow's milk daily and barely any solids at all. This leads to respiratory allergies, obe-

sity, iron-deficiency anemia, and, *not* least of all, elevated cholesterol levels due to the excess of saturated fat.

Calcium Balance and Bone Density

Recommendations published by the National Research Council's
Food and Nutrition Board indicate that at age 2 children need 800
mg of calcium; this increases to 1,200 mg by age 18. At best, these
are estimates, since many children of the world consume much less
than this but do not suffer calcium deficiencies. The amount of
calcium which finds its way from the food children consume into
their bones is offset to some degree by the calcium loss excreted
by the kidneys. The relationship between these two ongoing pro-
cesses is known as *calcium balance.* This determines *bone density:
the amount of calcium that remains in the bones.* Maximum bone
density is primarily developed during childhood, after which it is
intended to last a lifetime. Therefore, poor bone density established
during childhood and adolescence increases the risk of osteoporosis later in life.

Excessive protein in the child's diet increases calcium excretion
through the kidneys via a process whereby the protein causes acid-
ification of the urine. Children may absorb adequate amounts of
calcium from food, but then lose some of it through kidney excretion because of excessive protein in the diet. To avoid this, it's much
more sensible to obtain calcium from foods containing less protein
than milk and meat have.

Milk and Osteoporosis

Countries with the highest rates of osteoporosis, such as the United
States, England, and Sweden, consume the most milk. Dr. Mark
Hegsted, a former Harvard School of Public Health professor, said
in an interview for *Nutrition Action Healthletter* that countries like
China and Japan, where people eat much less protein and dairy
food, have low rates of osteoporosis.

The China Health Study (see Chapter 18) also showed that the rural Chinese, who consume less calcium than Americans, seem to have much less osteoporosis than do Americans, who drink milk throughout their childhood and, in most cases, throughout their lives.

Elderly South African Bantu women don't have osteoporosis, despite having a large calcium drain from nursing an average of 10 children. Their diet contains only about 440 mg of calcium, less than half what Americans consume. It appears that they are protected by their low intake of protein (50 grams daily, compared with 91 grams by Americans).

On the other hand, Eskimos consume a very high-protein diet (containing 250–400 grams daily) and consume far more calcium than Americans (2,000 mg daily); they also have one of the highest rates of osteoporosis in the world. According to a report in *Science* magazine in 1986, evidence is accumulating that calcium *intake* is not related to bone density. It seems that milk, with its excessive protein, *may be a part of the calcium problem instead of a solution.*

Cow's milk is high in calcium *and* protein, and therein lies the problem. Since only 28 percent of the calcium in dairy products is absorbed, and the excess protein promotes calcium excretion by the kidneys, milk and other dairy products may, over a lifetime, lead to severe deficiencies of calcium, and to osteoporosis.

We should consider nondairy sources of calcium, according to a letter to the editor of *The New York Times* by Dr. Neal Barnard, president of the Physicians' Committee for Responsible Medicine and an outspoken advocate of reducing fat and protein in children's diets. He was responding to an article of the previous week by health writer Jane Brody, who suggested low-fat milk as a good source of calcium. Dr. Barnard recommended instead green leafy vegetables, calcium-fortified orange juice, and legumes.

Almost all foods contain small portions of the calcium needed for an adequate diet. Collectively, these sources will provide enough calcium and not cause its loss through the kidneys, as does the excess protein found in dairy products. Many green vegetables are actually calcium-rich—a cup of spinach, for example, contains 500 mg.

Many of my colleagues insist that these nondairy foods contain inadequate amounts of calcium and that it isn't absorbed well. This is a widely believed myth, generally promoted by the dairy industry. Scientific findings that disprove it have often been disregarded.

A 1990 report in the *American Journal of Clinical Nutrition* concluded that greens such as kale and broccoli have very high levels of calcium. The report went on to say that the calcium in kale is absorbed at least as well as that in milk.

Milk Is Not the Best Calcium Source

Many nutritionists and dietitians have misjudged the quantity of calcium available from vegetables, because they have looked at calcium only in a given *weight* of food. This makes dairy products appear to be the richest source. The ideal diet of vegetables, fruits, grains, and legumes requires more food to produce the same number of calories as do smaller servings of meat, oils, and dairy products. Even proponents of dairy products are surprised when calcium is expressed as milligrams per 100 *calories.*

Calcium in Milligrams per 100 Calories

Arugula	1,300
Watercress	800
Turnip greens	650
Collard greens	548
Mustard greens	490
Spinach	450
Broccoli	387
Swiss cheese	250
Milk (2-percent)	245
Green onions	240

Calcium in Milligrams per 100 Calories (*cont.*)

Okra	213
Cabbage	196
Whole milk	190
Cheddar cheese	179
American cheese	160

Suddenly one sees that dairy products are *not* the best sources. This is very important, since any diet cannot meet nutritional requirements for good health without adequate calories. In other words, adequate amounts of vegetables, fruit, grains, and legumes are *better sources of calcium than meat and dairy products.* The reason is simple. Children on a meatless and dairyless diet usually consume adequate calories from a variety of vegetables just as their peers who eat meat and dairy products. Therefore, adequate calcium is easily consumed on an all-plant diet with few or no dairy products. This is why billions of people on earth who do not consume dairy products live healthy lives with a perfectly healthy calcium balance.

Milk Isn't Needed for Protein

It's clear that your child can get adequate calcium from nondairy sources, without consuming any dairy products. If he also eats no meat, you may naturally wonder whether he's getting enough protein. The answer is "yes" if he is on a plant-based diet with adequate calories that is also plentiful in vegetable proteins. As we have seen in the last chapter, protein from animal products is unnecessary and undesirable, because it coexists with fat and also carries with it an independent risk for heart disease and cancer.

The National Dairy Council has convinced many that milk and cheese are a necessary source of protein. They are a source of protein, but not without excess fat. Two ounces of Cheddar cheese may supply 14 grams of protein, but it also contains a whopping 18 grams of fat, 12 of them the dangerous saturated variety. More protein is contained in a serving of beans, which contain practically no fat at all.

Considering the strong evidence discussed above, milk is *not* necessary for calcium and protein. It may, in fact, when consumed during childhood—when bone density is being established—lead to a deficiency later in life. Nondairy, vegetable sources supply plenty of calcium without this added risk. As for protein, vegetable sources are more than adequate.

Chapter 8

Myth Eight:
Low-Fat Diets Lack
Vitamins and Minerals

When you eat more fruits and vegetables
to get more beta-carotine, you not only increase
your intake of the other antioxidants—C and E—
you also get other protective substances that have
not yet been fully studied.
> —*Annette B. Natow, Ph.D., R.D.*
> *Jo-Ann Heslin, M.A., R.D.*
> *The Antioxidant Vitamin Counter*

*V*ictoria Moran, author of "A Mom's Guide to Happy, Low-Fat Kids" (see Chapter 21), once wrote, "Plants are veritable vitamin factories." You'll never hear it expressed better than that. Remember this when well-meaning but misinformed friends and relatives tell you that your child's new meatless and dairyless diet may be deficient in these nutrients. Don't let *anyone* spoil your enthusiasm.

A low-fat diet *could* certainly be deficient in vitamins and minerals, if the calories from fat were not replaced with calories from vegetables, fruits, grains, and legumes. As I have discussed before, sufficient calories from these sources are the key to the ideal diet. Most authorities would agree that children eating the typical Western diet, consisting of meat and dairy products with insufficient vegetables and fruits, would be more likely to encounter vitamin and mineral deficiencies. Nutritionist Dr. Johanna Dwyer of Tufts University wrote in 1991 that in her opinion care must be taken with children between the ages of 2 and 5 to see that their mineral intake is sufficient. For older children, she wrote, the increase in fresh fruits and vegetables in the low-fat diet usually provides *more* minerals and vitamins than a diet full of fast food, potato chips, candy bars, pies, cakes, and ice cream.

Do Children Need Vitamin Supplements?

Thirteen vitamins are needed by humans. They are A, C, D, E, K, and eight B vitamins. All are obtained in adequate amounts from a variety of vegetables, fruits, whole grains, and legumes, except for vitamin B12, which is produced by bacteria in animals. Thus, children on a plant-based diet with adequate calories do not require supplemental vitamins, with the possible exception of vitamin B12.

Vitamin A is found in the form of beta carotene in leafy green vegetables, carrots, sweet potatoes, winter squash, and cantaloupe, in adequate amounts to supply a child's daily needs, which range from 1,000 IU at age 2 to 4,000 at age 18. One cup of any of these vegetables exceeds these requirements—a sweet potato or raw carrot supplies over 20,000 IU. As with all vitamins and minerals, the amount of vitamin A varies with the freshness of the vegetables and the cooking process—steaming is preferred.

Vitamin C, in adequate amounts for optimal health (ranging from 40 mg at age 2 to 60 mg at age 18), is found in citrus fruits, strawberries, green and leafy vegetables, cantaloupe, green pepper, cauliflower, potatoes, and sweet potatoes. One cup of green leafy vegetables or ½ cup of red, green, or yellow pepper exceeds these requirements, as does half a cantaloupe (which contains 112 mg).

The National Cancer Institute sent detailed food-diary questionnaires to 10,000 people and found that those on a low-fat diet get more of vitamins A and C and more fiber than those eating high-fat diets. Furthermore, those who ate the most fat consumed the fewest fruits, vegetables, and grains, and were the most likely to obtain insufficient vitamins and minerals. The questionnaires were completed by adults, but the information would apply equally to children.

Vitamin D may be consumed by eating all animal products, particularly sardines, herring, salmon, tuna, milk, egg yolk, and fish oils, but these are unnecessary, because it is also manufactured by the body on exposure to sunlight. Ten minutes of sunlight three times a week produces enough vitamin D to satisfy the body's daily needs—400 IU at all ages.

Vitamin E is easily consumed in adequate quantities without meat or dairy products. Excellent sources are nuts, seeds, and the vegetable oils of soybeans, cottonseed, sunflower, olives, and corn; but since these are all very high in fat, other plant sources should be eaten, such as wheat germ, corn, asparagus, spinach, broccoli, kale, Brussels sprouts, cucumber, whole-grain cereals, and enriched flour. Your child should eat a variety of these foods to reach the daily requirements of 6 IU at age 2 and up to 10 IU at age 18, since no single serving contains enough. The richest low-fat plant sources are kale and cucumber, containing 6 and 8 IU per cup, respectively.

Vitamins C, E, and beta carotene, which is converted by the body to vitamin A, are frequently called antioxidants. This trio has been the subject of intense scientific interest in recent years because of their apparent ability to prevent the oxidation of LDL. Oxidation, an ongoing metabolic process of this cholesterol-rich particle, enables it to invade arterial walls, as I discussed in Chapter 1. The antioxidant vitamins are therefore thought to be important in the prevention of heart disease. There is also evidence that they help prevent cancer. Vitamins C and E and beta carotene are obtained, according to the National Cancer Institute study mentioned above, in greater amounts by eating vegetables, fruits, and grains than from eating meat and dairy products. The daily requirements for these vitamins given above are only for preventing deficiencies; for their antioxidant effects, more may be needed. How much? Dr. JoAnn Manson, codirector of Women's Health at Harvard, suggested in an interview for *Family Circle* magazine that a daily total of 5 servings from a combination of fruits and vegetables would be enough. This is also the recommendation of the USDA Food Guide Pyramid—from the vegetable group, 3–5 servings; from the fruit group, 2–4 servings.

These vitamins alone, however, may not be effective in preventing heart disease and cancer when they are consumed as supplements. A 1994 study by the National Cancer Institute showed no protection from these diseases in 29,000 Finnish men taking these vitamins in the form of supplement tablets over eight years. A few months later a Dartmouth Medical School study showed that the same vitamin supplements for four years failed to prevent premalignant colon polyps in more than 800 subjects. There may be other substances in vegetables and fruit that offer the real protection seen in many studies for which these vitamins got the credit. According to a 1992 report, other substances, known as *phytochemicals,* present in fruits and vegetables, may be the *real* cancer protectors (see Chapter 13).

Vitamin K is necessary for normal blood-clotting, thereby preventing hemorrhages. Deficiencies are very rare (except in the newborn infant, who is routinely given an injection of vitamin K at the time of birth) since bacteria in the intestines manufacture 80 percent of the vitamin K the body needs, regardless of what foods are eaten. The remainder is easily obtained by eating a single serving of cabbage, cauliflower, spinach, or other leafy vegetables, or cereals, or soybean or other vegetable oils. Daily requirements are 0.015 mg at age 2, increasing to approximately 0.065 mg at age 18.

The B-Complex Vitamins

There is little disagreement among health authorities that vegetables and fruit are the best sources of vitamins A and C. Some, however, question whether plant-based foods supply adequate amounts of the B-complex vitamins. No clinical signs of nutritional deficiencies of these vitamins were found in the China Health Study (see Chapter 18) of the diets of 6,000 rural Chinese villagers eating, throughout their childhood, only vegetables, fruit, grains, and legumes. Furthermore, vegetarian children in Western countries who consume adequate calories from plant-based foods have not been found to develop B-complex deficiencies.

The B-complex vitamins are necessary for normal nerve, skeletal-muscle, and heart-muscle metabolism. There is a common opinion that B-complex vitamins also function best as a group rather than separately. The individual vitamins are obtained by eating a variety of vegetables, legumes, grains, and enriched cereals. Single servings of these foods usually supply less than the minimum daily needs, but collectively they are more than adequate. *It is unnecessary to count the amount of each vitamin supplied by each serving.*

The following B vitamins are adequately supplied by plant-based foods, with the exception of vitamin B12.

Vitamin B1 (thiamin) is found in brown rice, whole grains, peas, dried beans, soybeans, peanuts, fortified breads, pasta, and cereals. Fruits and vegetables are not high in B1, but when 5 daily servings are combined with 2 serving of grains or legumes, the daily requirement of 0.7 mg at age 2, and up to 1.5 mg at age 18, is easily satisfied. A single serving of Total Corn Flakes or Kellogg's Product 19 supplies 100 percent of your child's daily needs.

Vitamin B2 (riboflavin) is found in nuts, green, leafy vegetables, legumes, and fortified bread and cereal. Your child may consume his daily needs of 1 mg at age 2 to 1.3 mg at age 18 by eating a variety of these foods. The richest sources—whole-wheat pasta, wild rice, and the cereals Total Raisin Bran and Total Wheat Flakes—each supply your child's daily needs in a single serving.

Vitamin B3 (niacin) is supplied by whole-wheat bread, lentils, mushrooms, figs, dates, peanuts, brewer's yeast, and enriched bread and cereals. From these sources alone, children may obtain their daily needs of 9 mg at age 2 up to 20 mg at age 18. Here again, a variety of vegetables, fruits, and grains are needed. Total Corn Flakes supply 100 percent of your child's daily needs in one serving.

Vitamin B6 (pyridoxine) is available from bananas, cabbage, corn, oats, split peas, wheat bran, cantaloupe, and blackstrap molasses. A variety of these foods, along with almost any grain or a single serving of enriched cereal, is sufficient for the daily needs of 1 mg at age 2 up to 2 mg at age 18. Again, an enriched cereal such as Total Corn Flakes or Kellogg's Product 19 contains 100 percent of your child's daily needs in a single serving.

Folic acid, another B-complex vitamin, is important in the manufacture of DNA, which controls cell function. It also acts with B12 to produce red blood cells. The daily need is approximately 0.05 mg at age 2 up to 0.2 mg at age 18, which may be obtained by combining at least 5 servings from spinach, broccoli, turnip greens, whole grains, or fruits such as cantaloupe and strawberries. Single servings of several enriched cereals, such as Post Natural Bran Flakes and Total Corn Flakes, supply the total daily needs. In 1994, the FDA asked makers of bread and grains to add folic acid to all "enriched" products.

Now to the vitamin-B12 dilemma. For centuries, children in many parts of the world have been raised on low-fat diets with no ill effects. A single question remains for many nutritionists: can children eating no animal products whatsoever become deficient in vitamin B12? This is a legitimate concern, since B12 is found only in animal products. Therefore, for those worried about this, supplemental B12, contained in a multivitamin tablet, or nonfat milk— 1 cup of which contains double your child's daily B12 needs—may be consumed with breakfast cereals. Many cereals are also fortified with this vitamin. Tufts University nutritionist Johanna Dwyer suggests that rich sources are contained in B12-fortified soy milk and meat substitutes.

For some reason, not completely understood, vitamin-B12 deficiencies are rarely found in vegetarian children or adults consuming adequate calories from a vegetarian diet. Chinese children, for example, on a total vegetable, fruit, and grain diet show no symptoms attributable to deficiencies of vitamin B12. Furthermore, a little of this vitamin goes a long, long way. The body can store B12 for up to 5 years, so there is no need to consume it daily. Occasional supplies from skim milk and other nonfat dairy products, for instance, may be enough. The *average* daily needs are 0.001 mg for a 2-year-old up to 0.002 mg at age 18.

Biotin, another member of the B-complex group, is one of the few vitamins that can be totally produced by intestinal bacteria.

Children are *not* dependent on food for an adequate supply. It is found, however, in brown rice, nuts, fruits, and brewer's yeast. The daily requirement to prevent deficiency has been estimated to be 150 mg at age 2 and 300 mg at age 18, all of which may be synthesized in the intestines.

Vitamin B5 (pantothenic acid) may also be produced by the intestinal bacteria, but is also available from whole grains, bran, wheat germ, nuts, and green vegetables. Daily needs, all from internal synthesis, have been estimated to be 5 mg at age 2 and up to 10 mg at age 18.

Other B-complex vitamins have been identified, but very little is known of their sources and daily requirements. Those listed here represent the most important, according to current scientific knowledge.

Even though vitamin deficiencies are not usually found in children consuming adequate calories from a totally plant-based diet, I recommend that my patients on such a diet take a multivitamin tablet that includes B12 daily, unless they are eating fortified cereals or drinking nonfat milk. The vitamin supplement is the better choice, in my opinion, because of the potential allergies that may result from drinking milk or consuming it with cereals. Children in my clinic have found rice or soy milk substitutes to be palatable in dry cereals. Also, many instant "hot" cereals are prepared by adding hot water without milk.

Minerals

There are more than 60 minerals present in the human body, making up 4 percent of its weight. Only about 22 are considered essential, the most important being calcium, chlorine, magnesium, phosphorus, potassium, sodium, and sulfur. The remainder, called trace minerals, are present in minute amounts. All known minerals are available in sufficient amounts for good health from a variety of vegetables, fruit, whole grains, and legumes. Vegetable sources of calcium, for instance, as we have shown in the last chapter, are more than adequate.

I hope that any fears you may have had about vitamin and mineral deficiencies in a diet without meat or dairy products have been banished. Your child's low-fat diet—with the fat calories replaced by vegetables, fruits, grain, and legumes—supplies more vitamins and minerals than the food consumed by most of his playmates who eat meat and dairy products.

Chapter 9

Myth Nine:
A Low-Fat Diet Means
Limited Choices

Choices are relatively limited—and mostly fatty—at
the meat counter and the dairy case. But take a
walk through the produce section of your grocery
store, or stroll through a farmers' market. The sight
is a feast for the senses—so many different shapes,
sizes, aromas, textures, flavors, and colors.
—*Suzanne Havala, M.S., R.D.*

*"T*here's small choice in rotten apples," said Hortensio in *The Taming of the Shrew*. Similarly, many parents feel that when meat and dairy products are eliminated from a child's diet the remaining choices are severely limited—an impression given by those of us who have emphasized only the things that should be avoided. Parents often come up to me at seminars and ask, "What's left?"

Then I realize that I've stressed the things they *shouldn't* eat, without spending enough time discussing the variety of delicious foods compatible with good health. This would indeed be a limited diet if we advocated reducing fat without replacing its calories with a variety of vegetables, fruits, whole grains, and legumes. Food choices on a plant-based, low-fat diet are actually increased rather than decreased.

Only 10 Menus for Most

Dr. William Castelli, director of the Framingham Study, says that everyone should choose about 10 low-fat, high-complex-carbohydrate menus and stick to them. This is the average number of menus most people already use for their regular diets. The choices, however, from which these groups of food may be selected are enormous.

I now keep a prepared list of the variety of foods available to the child on a low-fat diet. My list starts with vegetables, since they are the most nutritionally rich. Most parents are stunned at the variety and never again ask about what to feed their children. In Chapter 21, "A Mom's Guide to Happy, Low-Fat Kids," professional food writer Victoria Moran offers tried-and-true methods for dealing with picky eaters, tips on getting your child to eat vegetables, fruits, and grains, and suggested menus for low-fat meals at home.

Vegetables

The following are, according to the U.S. Department of Agriculture, the 20 most commonly consumed vegetables: potatoes, iceberg lettuce, tomatoes, onions, carrots, celery, sweet corn, broccoli, green cabbage, cucumbers, bell peppers, cauliflower, leaf lettuce, sweet potatoes, mushrooms, onions, green beans, radishes, summer squash, and asparagus.

If this isn't enough to choose from, consider artichokes, eggplant, chicory, collard greens, kale, kohlrabi, leeks, jalapeño peppers, rhubarb, beets, Brussels sprouts, garlic, mustard greens, okra, spinach, turnips, parsley, shallots, and squashes.

Most of these vegetables are grown in many varieties. For example, the summer squashes (yellow straightneck, yellow crookneck, zucchini, golden zucchini, baby, chayote, and pattypan) and the winter squashes (acorn, golden acorn, table queen, pumpkin, banana, spaghetti, delicata, turban, butternut, sweet dumpling, buttercup, golden nugget, and hubbard) offer 20 distinctly different varieties of a single vegetable family.

"And the Winner Is . . . !"

*N*utrition Action Healthletter, published by the Center for Science in the Public Interest, rated 58 vegetables in October 1993, based on their nutrients and fiber content. The winner by a large margin was the sweet potato, followed by the raw carrot. The sweet potato, eaten less frequently than most green vegetables and legumes (see the chart on page 106), remains a favorite with most nutritionists. It was praised by the *University of Texas Lifetime Health Letter*. They called it a "nutritional bonanza," rich in vitamins A, C, and B6, copper, potassium, riboflavin, and beta carotene. Sweet potatoes are also rich in fiber. Also high on the *Nutrition Action Healthletter* list were broccoli, Brussels sprouts, and squash. These are the best, and the most nutritionally dense, but it's impossible to find a bad fresh vegetable. Frozen or canned products are acceptable alternates if freshness is questionable.

Fruit

*T*he USDA lists the 20 most commonly consumed fruits as bananas, apples, watermelons, oranges, cantaloupe, grapes, grapefruit, strawberries, peaches, pears, nectarines, honeydew melons, plums, avocados, lemons, pineapples, tangerines, sweet cherries, kiwi fruit, and lime. Other choices include apricots, kumquats, cherimoya, starfruit, blackberries, raspberries, blueberries, cranberries, plantains, dates, figs, mangoes, papayas, persimmons, and pomegranates. Nearly all of these 35 fruits are available in a dried form. The color and variety are voluminous.

Modern methods for harvesting, shipping, and storing have made fresh fruit available to almost anyone at any time of the year. Their attraction for children is their sweet taste, but nutritionally most fruits are rich in vitamins, especially vitamin C and beta carotene, the precursor of vitamin A. Fruits are also very low in fat and high in fiber. Avocados should be avoided, however; they contain about as much total fat as beef and are also moderately high in saturated fat. Concentrated fruit is commonly used for taste enhancement in low- and non-fat snacks.

Both vegetables and fruits are now available in a variety of hybrids. Broccoflower, tiny bite-sized kiwi, and heads of lettuce the size of tennis balls are among dozens of these genetically engineered items appearing during the 1990s. The varieties will undoubtedly continue to multiply. The first genetically engineered tomato, with a longer shelf life, was approved by the FDA in 1994. You can expect many more genetically altered vegetables.

Whole Grains

Whole grains are readily available to the consumer in a wide variety of preparations such as pasta, bread, flour, and cereal. Individual whole grains include wheat, rye, corn, rice, barley, oats, and millet. Some of the other selections from a total of 30 varieties of grains are wild rice, spelt, amaranth, quinoa, and kasha. Refined grains are not as desirable, since they contain less fiber, fewer vitamins and minerals, and more calories. But even refined grains, which are often fortified with these nutrients, are preferable to high-fat, high-protein meat and dairy products.

Grains are neglected by consumers in most Western countries. For example, they contribute 25 percent of calories in the United States, compared with 65 percent of calories in Japan, India, and China. These countries have found a wide variety of uses for grains, because their longer shelf life makes them more available than either vegetables or fruit. With the exception of oats and oat bran— both are excellent low-fat choices, although slightly higher in fat than the others—grains will keep almost indefinitely if frozen. The higher fat content of oats and oat bran cause them to turn rancid after only two or three months in the freezer.

Legumes

Commonly consumed legumes are dozens of varieties of beans and peas, including black beans, pinto beans, kidney beans, lima beans, Great Northern beans, navy beans, soybeans, black-eyed peas, split green peas, yellow peas, chick-peas, lentils, mung beans, fava beans, and cranberry beans. Legumes contain more protein than any other plant food. As a source of fiber, legumes are second only to wheat bran. They are also very low in fat, inexpensive, and versatile.

Legumes are available in dried form but are also widely available canned, requiring no soaking or cooking. They may be eaten separately or used in casseroles, soups, salads, and sandwiches. Legumes are also a low-fat ingredient for dips.

A Plant-Based Diet Means Variety

So, if you're worrying that a meatless and dairyless diet may limit your child's choices, be reassured that the only limitations are animal proteins, fats, and oils. Children on a meatless and dairyless diet, by definition, eat a greater variety of foods than do typical meat- and dairy-eaters. And your child is not likely to run out of new vegetables and fruits to sample.

Chapter 10

Myth Ten:
Low-Fat Diets Retard Growth

"Please test your servants for ten days: Give us
nothing but vegetables to eat and water to drink.
Then compare our appearance with that of the
young men who eat the royal food, and treat your
servants in accordance with what you see." So he
agreed to this and tested them for ten days.

At the end of the ten days they looked healthier
and better nourished than any of the young men
who ate the royal food. So the guard took away
their choice food and the wine they were to drink
and gave them vegetables instead.

—*Daniel 1:12–16*

*T*here seems to be some lingering doubt among health authorities—chiefly the NIH and the AAP—whether children consuming a diet sufficiently low in fat to prevent heart disease and cancer
will grow to their full potential adult height. This feeling has
emerged because of surveys which included malnourished children
eating low-fat diets *without* sufficient calories, carbohydrates, vitamins, or minerals. Entirely different results were found when the
children studied were on a purposeful, supervised low-fat diet with
adequate calories.

In January 1992, after reviewing all available scientific evidence, the Department of Community and Family Medicine at the University of California at San Diego concluded that the studies reporting growth retardation of children on low-fat diets were seriously flawed, that any effect on growth would be very small. Some of these reports, discussed below, showed *greater* growth on low-fat vegetarian diets. *Children on low-fat diets of mostly vegetables, fruits, grain, and legumes, when consuming adequate calories, not only grow normally, but have actually been shown to attain greater height than meat-eating children.*

For more than 40 years, studies of Seventh-Day Adventist children and their parents, who had been on meatless diets since childhood, have shown no evidence of growth retardation. These studies are not tainted by the inclusion of malnourished children.

Loma Linda University compared the growth of 1,765 California children attending state schools and Seventh-Day Adventist schools. In their report of January 1991, the Seventh-Day Adventist students, who ate far less meat but much more vegetables and fruits than the state school children, attained a *greater* height. This study concluded that low-fat diets with an abundance of vegetables, fruits, and grains carried no risk of growth retardation.

The authors of the Loma Linda Study published another report, in the *Journal of the American Dietetic Association* in 1992, which showed that vegetarian children were more likely to enter a natural period of slower growth during adolescence than meat-eating children. This slow growth period did not affect ultimate height. Vegetarian children and adolescents who consumed a nutritionally balanced diet grew at least as tall as, if not taller than, nonvegetarian children.

A survey of children purposely placed on low-fat balanced diets was studied by Arizona pediatricians Drs. Friedman and Goldberg. They carefully followed 51 infants on a low-fat, plant-based diet to the age of 3. These children maintained the same growth rate in length, weight, and head size as a control group of 420 children fed a typical American diet. The only difference found in the two groups was a much lower cholesterol level in the low-fat group.

There is a well-known community-based study of children whose parents had purposefully chosen a low-fat but nutrition-rich diet for their children. That community, known as "The Farm," was established in rural central Tennessee in 1971.

The Farm Study

The Farm Study, done by the Centers for Disease Control's Division of Nutrition, was reported in the journal *Pediatrics* in 1989. The growth of 404 vegetarian children in this planned community of vegetarians was found to be essentially the same as standard growth patterns in the United States.

Eighty-three percent of these children had been strict vegetarians since birth, eating no animal products at all. By the age of 10, the vegetarian children attained a height and weight equal to the normal values for children of that age in the United States published by the National Center for Health Statistics. This is another of the untainted studies excluding neglected and malnourished children.

These findings should not come as a surprise, since you now know that a diet of vegetables, fruit, grains, and legumes contains more of the vitamins, minerals, fiber, and plant protein necessary for full growth than the typical Western meat-based diet. The key here is adequate calories, so you may feel more secure with some knowledge of the caloric needs for full growth. The following guideline is included only to satisfy your academic curiosity, since children on unlimited portions of vegetables, fruits, and grains will naturally eat enough food to obtain enough calories.

A good rule of thumb to follow in order to make sure your child is getting adequate calories is to supply 40 calories per inch of height for a child between 1 and 3 years of age. For example, a 2-year-old measuring 30 inches would require approximately 1,200 calories daily. For children between the ages of 4 and 10, you may estimate needed calories by multiplying their weight by 36. Thus, a typical 10-year-old girl weighs 70 pounds, and needs approximately 2,100 calories daily. Children's caloric needs vary widely, depending on their physical activity and rate of growth. Once these estimates are made and you are reassured, forget about counting calories.

Considering the Adolescent "Growth Spurt"

Older children and adolescents on reduced-fat diets also show no signs of growth retardation. Seventeen-year-olds in Turkey, Greece, and Israel who consume 30–35 percent of their calories as fat were compared with American 17-year-olds who consume more than 50 percent of their calories as fat. No difference was found in the adolescent growth period between the two groups. The average height of Israeli boys and girls for the ages of 15 through 19 is the same as that of Americans.

These studies have given us reasons to expect normal growth in children on low-fat diets, but for those who need more proof, a long-term intervention study by the NIH is now under way. The Dietary Intervention Study in Children (DISC) is designed to study the growth and school performance of 9- and 10-year-old boys and 8- and 9-year-old girls with high cholesterol levels as they progress through the rapid-growth adolescent years.

Half of the children will be placed on a low-fat diet of which 28 percent of the calories come from total fat, 8 percent from saturated fat, and less than 150 mg a day of cholesterol—not low enough in fat to control cholesterol levels and prevent coronary heart disease. The other half will consume a typical American diet. The DISC's intent is to determine once and for all if a "low-fat" diet contains enough minerals, vitamins, and protein. Early data in 1995 shows normal growth.

However, while we wait for this "proof"—the study could take a decade or more—another generation of children will enter adulthood with coronary heart disease and die prematurely. This is reminiscent of the early 1950s, when Dr. Ernst Wynder insisted that we already had enough evidence that cigarette smoking caused cancer. Millions more died of the disease while medical authorities and the tobacco companies waited for more proof. Today the National Beef Industry Council and the National Dairy Council have replaced the tobacco companies in this scenario.

The late Dr. Alton Oschner, founder of the famed Oschner Clinic in New Orleans, agreed with Dr. Wynder's warnings at that time. He told me the following parable at a conference: "Natasha suspected that Ivan, her husband, was unfaithful to her. One evening she followed him to a cottage, where he was received by a beautiful young woman inside. Through the window, Natasha could see them embracing, disrobing, and approaching the bedroom. As the light went off, Natasha said to herself, 'If I only had proof.' "

Do Meat and Dairy Products Retard Growth?

The National Beef Industry Council and the National Dairy Council may have to take the defensive on the growth issue. Until recently, no one considered the possibility that excessive consumption of meat and dairy products may lead to growth retardation. Early menarche in girls, accompanied by early closure of growth centers in their long bones, which slows and finally arrests growth, is common in meat-eating societies. Usually, growth in height ceases within 1 to 1½ years after the onset of menstruation. This may reduce final adult height.

More scientists are now stating publicly that a low-fat diet is not only safe for children, but almost certainly more healthful than the present typical American children's diet.

For example, Dr. Peter O. Kwiterovich, Jr., chief of the Lipid Research and Atherosclerosis Unit at the Johns Hopkins University School of Medicine, has written in his book *The Johns Hopkins Complete Guide for Preventing and Reversing Heart Disease* that he has found no rational basis for thinking that a low-fat diet may adversely affect the growth and development of children. He says, "Some argue that the brain needs cholesterol to grow. But by the age of two years 90 percent of brain growth is completed. The brain and other organs in the child can manufacture as much cholesterol as is needed without saturated fat."

Based on the studies that I have discussed above, it appears that children on low-fat diets with adequate calories grow normally—although probably at a somewhat slower rate—and reach full adult height. Children on high-fat diets grow faster, but develop more chronic diseases and have a shorter life span.

This slower growth may be the norm for both humans and animals who experience optimal health and have the longest life span. French biologist Charles Buffon found that most animals tend to live six times their period of growth. Slower growth to maturity always predicted longer life spans. This, applied to the human species, would seem to confirm that the slower growth to maturity on a low-fat diet would lead to a longer life span. The longer period of growth, seen among vegetarian children to near the age of 17 or 18, would, by this formula, be compatible with a maximum life span of 102 to 108 years.

Chinese Children Grow on Vegetables and Grains

Dr. T. Colin Campbell, director of the China Health Study, insists that full adult height is attained on a diet based totally on plant foods. There has been a dramatic increase in adult height among the Chinese during the 1953–82 period, when the rural Chinese children consumed more calories from plant protein but without increases in animal protein. It was childhood infections, he says, that caused the growth retardation in Chinese children. He concludes that attaining full body height, even in less industrialized countries, can be obtained with the consumption of a plant-rich diet, if it is adequate in amount, quality, and variety.

A related concern of parents, that children on a low-fat diet will lack energy, is also unfounded. High-energy foods are complex carbohydrates, not fat. Exercise physiologists have found that athletic performance is enhanced by complex carbohydrates to a greater degree than by either fat or protein.

Chapter 11

Myth Eleven:
It's Obvious Which Foods
Are High in Fat

A silent predator lurking there,
Like a lion in the bush, waiting.
—*Lauren Vice, sixth grade,*
Academy of the Sacred Heart
Grand Coteau, Louisiana

*W*hen counseling the family of a child with a high blood-cholesterol level, I first discuss the obvious sources of saturated fat, such as meat, dairy products, butter, and cooking oils. At this point, the child's parents are usually one step ahead of me. They have often *already* reduced or even discontinued them, only to find, after three months, that their child's cholesterol level is still high. There are still "predators in the bush"; so now our serious work begins: to teach the family about hidden fat.

Hillary Clinton was so concerned about the high-fat foods served in the White House that she invited Dr. Dean Ornish to come and teach the White House cooks, including chef Pierre Chambrin, how to reduce the fat in their meals. This required a knowledge of where the fat was found, so Dr. Ornish conducted "in–White House" seminars to help the staff identify unexpected sources of fat in various types of food. The First Family's position was well publicized in the media, boosting the awareness of hidden dietary fat among millions of Americans who had not thought much about it before. Chambrin ignored Dr. Ornish's advice and went ahead with his high-fat French cooking, explaining that *he* must decide how he cooked. "I have a different concept of food," he said to a *USA Today* reporter. He and his staff were fired a few months later and replaced by Walter S. Scheib III, recruited from the Greenbrier Resort and Health Spa, who readily agreed to consult with Dr. Ornish about hidden fats. The new first chef isn't likely to banish all fat from the first family and staff. *Harper's* magazine reported in "Harper's Index" (April 1994) that the White House Domino's Pizza orders increased by 18 percent each day when Hillary Clinton was out of town.

From the White House to Our House

In my seminars I use the acronym "M-E-D-I-C-S" to teach physicians and their patients where they should look for unexpected sources of fat. You may also find it helpful in planning meals for your child. "M" is for "meat," "E" for "eggs," "D" for "dairy products," "I" for "invisible fat," "C" for "condiments," and "S" for "snacks." It's very easy to remember and will help you organize your fat-search.

Meat

The saturated fat and total fat in meat are obvious to most people. Although the beef industry has strongly promoted "low-fat cuts," it would be difficult to find any cut of meat that did not derive at least 40 percent of its calories from fat. Furthermore, the majority of fat in meat is saturated and raises blood-cholesterol levels.

The white, skinless meat of poultry and fish contains far less total and saturated fat than beef but no less animal protein, which, as already discussed, raises cholesterol levels and increases the risk of coronary heart disease.

Eggs

Eggs, relatively high in cholesterol, contain only 1.7 grams of saturated fat each. This is the reason several studies have reported that 3 to 5 eggs per week may be acceptable for a low-fat diet for all but strict vegetarians. However, the 1.7 grams of saturated fat become significant if you eat a 3- or 4-egg omelette. As for cholesterol, improved analytical methods have revised the egg-yolk content downward, from 274 mg to between 213 and 220 mg. Based on this, the AHA has revised its suggested maximum consumption of whole eggs from 3 to 4 per week.

For the omelette-lover, there are fat-free and cholesterol-free products, such as Scramblers, Egg Beaters, Omlette Mix, and Second Nature, which are ready for cooking. Egg whites are also fat- and cholesterol-free. In most recipes, 2 egg whites can be substituted for each whole egg. Also, there are whole-egg products ready for the cooking pan which have the usual yolk cholesterol reduced from 220 to 45 mg. One such product, Simply Eggs (Michael Foods, Inc.), is made by centrifuging the yolks, which separates out some of the cholesterol. Practically *all* cholesterol is removed by extraction with solvents in products expected to reach the market during the mid-1990s.

Dairy

Dairy products, except for skim milk and its derivatives, are also dangerously high in saturated fat. Even so-called low-fat (2-percent) milk derives 35 percent of its calories from fat. A 7-ounce glass of whole milk contains 8 grams of fat and 4 grams of saturated fat. Skim milk and buttermilk are the lowest-fat alternatives; each contains less than 1 gram of saturated fat per serving. Although these are essentially nonfat foods, it must be remembered that they, along with products made from them, contain the same amount of animal protein as all other dairy products.

Invisible Fat

Saturated fat is found in unexpected places, where children get a large portion of the excess fat in their diets. Once you have learned where to look for them, they are easily recognized. A child over the age of 5 may learn to identify foods that harbor hidden fat and the reasons for avoiding such foods.

When your child has reduced, discontinued, or replaced the meat and dairy products in her diet, you must then turn your attention to her other sources of fat, such as candy, cookies, and pastries. These items are often thought of as "sweets" but may contain highly saturated vegetable oils. Avocados, olives, and nuts, including coconuts, are other unexpected sources of fat. In my seminars, I refer to these foods as containing "invisible fats." A Hershey Golden Almond bar, for example, contains 11 grams of fat, including 5 grams of saturated fat. A sugar-coated doughnut contains 9.5 grams of fat, including 4.3 grams of saturated fat. As an alternative, a fig bar contains only 1 gram of total fat and ½ gram of saturated fat.

You must ferret out most of the foods containing invisible fat and select alternatives. Some foods are designated by names that falsely imply that the item is very low in fat, whereas they may be high in the fat contained in vegetable oils. Many brands of granola, for example, contain nearly 5 grams of fat per serving, including 3.3 grams of saturated fat. Grape-Nuts, on the other hand, is fat-free. Another example would be a bran muffin, containing 5 grams of fat, whereas a plain bagel or an English muffin each contains only 1 gram of fat.

Condiments

Condiments have also enjoyed the reputation of being low in fat. Unfortunately, many low-fat foods are converted into very high-fat servings by the addition of high-fat condiments. Examples are sour cream, mayonnaise, salad dressings, butter, gravies, and sauces. All are available in low-fat or fat-free versions, usually identified by the word "lite," but it's important to read the label to be sure.

Low-fat vegetable sauces can be made at home by a method

created by Jerry Edwards of Chef's Expressions Catering in Timonium, Maryland. He uses a juicer to reduce the vegetables—root vegetables such as beets, carrots, and turnips work best—to liquid. The vegetable is then placed in a sauté pan on a low burner to thicken while you are whipping into it "slurry," a soupy paste made of arrowroot. "It's all done very quickly," he said in a *Baltimore Sun* interview. "The key to these sauces is to stop cooking them when they get to their brightest color."

A homemade substitute for sour cream is low-fat or nonfat yogurt with lemon juice. Mustard and ketchup are fat-free condiments that may be used to enhance a food's acceptance by children. Ketchup in usual servings supplies only 6 percent of the daily requirements for sodium, whereas Hunt's No Salt Added and Westbrae's low-salt ketchup are practically sodium-free. Usual servings of mustard supply approximately 2–5 percent of a child's daily sodium requirement. Salt from the shaker in moderation is an acceptable condiment. The majority of excess sodium in children's diets is within the food, naturally or added during cooking. Only about 15 percent comes from the salt added to the surface of the food before eating. These fat-free condiments may be your child's best enticement for eating vegetables during the early days of their new diet. I would suggest not exceeding the usual serving sizes printed on the labels. Tomato sauce, however, must be watched. Often thought to be nearly fat-free, it may contain large amounts of oil. All sauces may be added to food sparingly to reduce fat when a fat-free version isn't available. If you are eating out, insist that sauces be served on the side.

Snacks

Foods consumed between meals may be very high in saturated and total fat. The word "bran" is often misleadingly used in snack-product names. Again, bran muffins are touted as a low-fat snack with the added value of oat bran, a soluble fiber known to reduce cholesterol levels. But most bran muffins are low in bran and high in fat, which supplies more than 50 percent of their calories.

Most packaged cookies, candy, and chips are unacceptably high in total and saturated fat. Many of these have coconut oil or palm oil, which extends shelf life but is dangerously high in saturated fat. Beware of most theater popcorn, which is popped in coconut oil. A medium bag of 16 cups of buttered popcorn from six theater chains in three cities, analyzed by the Center for Science in the Public Interest, contained 56 grams of fat—most of it saturated—which is more than a bacon-and-eggs breakfast, a Big Mac and fries for lunch, and a steak dinner, all combined. Without the added butter, it still had 43 grams. A typical small bag contained 20 grams of total fat and 14 grams of saturated fat (exceeding a full day's healthy allotment for most children). Within a few weeks of the survey most large theater chains offered their customers a choice of regular or fat-free air-popped popcorn. Others switched from coconut oil to hydrogenated canola oil.

Low-Fat Snacks You Can Count On

Examples of truly low-fat snacks are plain bagels, English muffins, fruit, pretzels, graham crackers, vanilla wafers, fat-free yogurt, raisin bread, rice cakes, raw vegetable sticks, and air-popped popcorn. Microwave popcorn usually has between 5 and 10 grams of fat in each 3-cup serving. There are exceptions: Weaver Light has only 1 gram of fat per 3-cup serving, and 2 grams of fiber.

Fat-free cookies almost always have their taste enhanced by *concentrated fruit;* for this reason, they are often unexpectedly high in calories. Though it's practically impossible to consume too many calories on a low-fat diet of fresh vegetables, fruits, grains, and legumes, calories do become a problem with many of the fat-free snacks now sold in the supermarkets. For example, fat-free Fig Newtons contain 70 calories each, and it's a rare child who eats just one. Low-fat cookies—Oreos, for example—usually contain only about 20 percent less fat than the regular variety. Other packaged snacks are keeping their high-fat content, just adding vitamins.

If you get into the habit of using my acronym "M-E-D-I-C-S," invisible fat will probably not be overlooked in your child's diet. Once the sources are identified, they are usually never forgotten.

Chapter 12

Myth Twelve:
No One Knows What's
Really Best for My Child

To become properly acquainted with a
truth we must first have disbelieved it, and
disputed against it.
　　　—Prince Otto von Bismark (1815–98)
　　　　Prussian statesman

*E*arlier, I said that books such as mine share bookstore-shelf
space with volumes that are not based on scientific findings. Some
of them would have you feed your children *more,* not less, animal
fats and dairy products. Why should you, the reader, find what I
say more credible than books advocating supplements, megavita-
mins, amino acids, and high-protein diets?

When asked, I often tell people that my specialty in medicine is
children's nutrition, and that I have found the answer to preventing
the leading causes of death when children grow up. This always
gets their attention. What, they ask themselves, has he discovered?

After I explain the relationship between children's dietary fat and
high blood cholesterol, and heart disease and cancer when they
become adults, they are usually still skeptical. "Well, what do *you*
think we should feed them?" they usually ask without much enthu-

siasm. Then I say that children should consume less fat and more carbohydrates and fiber, and add that these changes can be achieved only by avoiding meat and dairy products and replacing them with plentiful amounts of vegetables, fruit, whole grains, and legumes. I've learned to expect a sigh and a roll of the eyes.

Who can blame them? How can anyone read the newspapers, watch TV, or browse the bookstores without total confusion? It appears that the experts do nothing but contradict one another. Does anyone really know the right answers?

"Planned" Confusion

First of all, there are massive lobbying efforts by the beef and dairy industries. The free teaching guides supplied by them to teachers when most of you were in grade school left an indelible perception that meat and dairy products are an indispensable source of calcium, protein, iron, and vitamins. This one misguided perception has thrown a million facts out the window, and we have literally ignored a half-century of proof that the typical Western diet during childhood is shortening our children's lives. The same lobbying has been similarly effective with the health agencies of the federal government.

The Certified Facts

The fact is that careful scientific studies, conducted by university centers and government agencies, have all come to the same conclusion. There can no longer be any room for doubt that children eat too much fat, not enough complex carbohydrates, and far too little fiber.

When the first large clinical studies, the Multiple Risk Factor Intervention Trial, commonly known as MRFIT—where dietary fat was reduced, comparing control and study groups—began publishing its reports in 1982, and the Helsinki Heart Study—where the effects of lowering cholesterol levels with drugs was studied—was reported in 1987, the dietary fat–cholesterol–heart-disease connection was conclusively proved. By 1987, the media seemed to be writing incessantly about the evils of dietary fat.

Unfortunately, this healthful momentum would be broken. In 1989, T. J. Moore wrote "The Cholesterol Myth," which was published in *The Atlantic* as a 33-page excerpt from his book *Heart Failure*, and has been widely quoted to this day. Moore, with no scientific training, seemed to convince many reporters across the country that dietary intervention had little effect on heart disease. Among other things, Moore used early reports of the MRFIT studies, which had shown less-than-expected reductions in heart disease— because the control groups voluntarily reduced their fat to near that of the study groups—to make a convincing argument that reducing dietary fat doesn't prevent heart disease. He was outmatched in a radio debate with Dr. William Castelli in 1991, but the magazine article is still being used by some to suggest that a low-fat diet is futile.

So You Want Proof?

By 1958 in this country (see Chapter 18), and as early as 1930 in Europe, absolute proof was found that coronary-artery disease begins during childhood. When autopsy studies revealed coronary-artery lesions in children only in countries where adults had coronary disease and where both children and adults consumed a high-fat diet and had high cholesterol levels, there was little doubt left that high-fat diets caused coronary disease in children. But more evidence was to come.

Finally, several studies (some as long as 20 years) of individual children revealed that those consuming high-fat diets had high cholesterol levels and developed coronary-artery lesions. These were found at autopsies of children who died unexpectedly of other causes (see Chapter 18). The children with the highest-fat diets had the highest cholesterol levels and the greatest number of coronary-artery lesions.

This was all the proof I needed after watching the evidence come in over a 20-year period. The public, however, remained confused by the dozens of media reports by poorly informed writers, which began appearing during the early 1990s (some continued to use the article in *The Atlantic* as a reference). Many of these media reports were based on misunderstandings of the scientific facts. Some were based on sincere opinions unfortunately influenced by the dairy and beef industries, or in some cases by pharmaceutical companies who make cholesterol-lowering drugs, as will be discussed later.

The facts are conclusive. Part Three of this book is designed to give you better insight into the studies and investigations that should have a profound impact upon your child's health and life span. Decide for yourself.

Part Two

Feeding Children
in the Real World

Practical Approaches

• • •

When we save our children, we save ourselves.
—*Margaret Mead*
(1901–78)

Chapter 13

4 Stages to an Ideal Diet

Some habits must be eased downstairs
a step at a time.

—*Mark Twain*
(1835–1910)

*T*o achieve an ideal diet with only 10–15 percent of its calories
derived from fat, one has to be very selective about snacks, meat,
and dairy products. However, reducing dietary fat this much isn't
difficult if approached gradually in stages. The saturated fat in such
a diet is quite low, only 3–5 percent of calories, and does not need
to be calculated, since there's very little in the foods your child will
be eating.

This is not the "moderate" diet with portions from *all* food
groups, including meat, milk, and oils—as recommended by the
U.S. Department of Agriculture's arbitrary "Pyramid"—which was
designed to be a politically satisfying guideline to please the country's powerful agribusiness.

As already discussed, "moderation" in America and other Western
nations involves eating high-fat foods and causes coronary heart
disease, hypertension, stroke, obesity, and diabetes. More *extreme*
measures are needed to prevent these diseases. They are not to be
taken lightly. "Tell a man whose house is on fire to give a moderate
alarm; tell him to moderately rescue his wife from the hands of the
ravisher; tell the mother to gradually extricate her babe from the

fire into which it has fallen; but urge me not to use moderation in a case like the present," wrote W. L. Garrison, an American abolitionist, during the early nineteenth century.

Cold Turkey?

So how do you begin to change your child's diet to reach the desirable 10–15 percent of calories from fat? Dr. Dean Ornish believes that it's easier to eliminate meat, poultry, fish, cheese, and other high-fat foods *entirely* than to cut back on them. Your palate, he says, never gets a chance to readjust if you keep eating meat, even in smaller quantities, because eating a little only makes you want more.

This "sudden" approach has certainly worked for the adults on the Ornish Program. But keep in mind that these are adults, and sick adults at that. They already have severe coronary disease in most cases. When making dietary changes in healthy children, you will probably find that a gradual approach works best.

Dr. T. Colin Campbell of Cornell University and Dr. Neal Barnard of George Washington University have independently suggested that the ideal diet should be reached in stages, each lasting several weeks. In my clinic, patients make the adjustments in 4 stages. Patients require 3 to 6 weeks at each stage to establish new eating habits, depending on the individual. I have discussed, in Chapter 3, studies which show that changing the fat taste may take up to 12 weeks, so there is no rush to move from one stage to the next.

Making the Transition

My plan, "4 Stages to an Ideal Diet," should not be confused with the AHA Step I and Step II diet recommendation (see page 103) for adults at moderate or high risk for heart disease. The 4 stages are intended to be just that, *transitional stages* for your child, to help him reach the ideal diet. While he is going through the 4 stages, it isn't necessary to count calories from fat or grams of fat consumed.

Just follow the guidelines listed below and your child will consume the correct amount of fat for each stage.

Stage 1

Stage 1 is actually comparable to the Step I diet recommended by the AHA, in which up to 30 percent of calories from fat are allowed. Your child may reach this level by simply limiting meat to 3 ounces (trimmed and cooked) daily, substituting low-fat (1 percent) or skim milk for whole milk, substituting low-fat dairy products for those made from whole milk, avoiding fried foods, and limiting desserts and snacks to no more than 1 a day. The calories reduced by these changes should be replaced by increasing the consumption of vegetables, fruits, grains, and legumes. She may eat as much of these foods as she desires, without limits.

As already discussed, this degree of fat reduction—as in the current national guidelines—is not enough to reduce the blood-cholesterol level sufficiently to prevent coronary heart disease or cancer. Therefore, it should be considered only as a transition for your child, for the first 3 to 12 weeks.

Stage 2

Stage 2 allows only 20–25 percent of calories from fat, much less than the NIH and AHA Step II diet (30 percent of calories from total fat and 7 percent from saturated fat), which was designed for adults at high risk. To achieve my Stage 2 level, your child should eat 3 ounces or less of trimmed lean meat, skinless breast of turkey or chicken, or fish no more than three times a week. Poultry and fish are lower in fat than beef, but contain almost as much animal protein. They are, along with lean meat, acceptable at Stage 2, but are further limited in the next stage. Fried foods are to be avoided, and cooking oils should be limited to those containing very little saturated fat, such as canola oil.

While in Stage 2, your child may drink skim milk and use fat-free dairy products. Low-fat or nonfat desserts and snacks should be limited to one a day. Suggestions for these are found in Chapter 22. Many nonfat snacks, as already discussed, are relatively high in calories because they have a base of concentrated fruit. The remainder of Stage 2 consists of vegetables, fruits, grains, and legumes in unlimited amounts. This stage represents a more healthful diet than Stage 1, but since it maintains the "fat taste," and many children continue to have elevated cholesterol levels on such a diet, it still falls short of ideal.

Stage 3

Stage 3 requires that trimmed lean meat, skinless turkey or chicken breast, and fish be eaten only occasionally (a maximum of once a week) or used only sparingly, as if they were condiments, with a diet of vegetables, fruits, grains, and legumes. For example, a dish of plain pasta topped with steamed vegetables may have small bits of crabmeat or shrimp added as a final "condiment." Small cubes of ham could also be added to such a dish. Nonsoy, fat-free meat substitutes are considered as vegetables (such as the Garden-Veggie, Garden-Mexi, and Garden-Sausage sold by Wholesome and Hearty Foods; see page 117); the soy variety contains excessive fat and sodium. Fried foods and cooking oils (except spray-on Pam) are avoided. Only nonfat milk and dairy products are allowed. Fat-free desserts or snacks may be eaten once a day.

Stage 3 allows 15–20 percent of calories from fat, which is adequate to reduce cholesterol levels sufficiently to prevent heart disease and fat-related cancer, but it too maintains the child's "fat taste." Therefore, to achieve the ideal plant-based diet for your child, you should proceed to Stage 4. Menus and recipes for Stage 4 are found in Chapters 22 and 23.

Stage 4

The ideal diet for your child consists of *vegetables, fruits, grains, and legumes in unlimited quantities;* this includes nonsoy fat-free meat substitutes. Nonfat dairy products and egg whites are allowed, but unnecessary. Children with allergies should avoid them. It isn't necessary to count calories, grams of fat, or grams of saturated fat. This diet derives less than 15 percent of its calories from total fat, and only 3–5 percent from saturated fat. Poultry and fish are *not* included here, because of their fat and animal-protein content. Soon the fat taste will be lost and your child will relish these foods in their endless varieties. Vitamin B12 sources or supplements are recommended for children in Stage 4 (see page 76).

As I have discussed before, you have nothing to fear about vitamin and mineral deficiencies, and your child will grow normally and reach her full adult height. It is estimated that 75 percent of the world's children thrive on this diet. Comparable to the rural Chinese and Japanese diet, it derives no more than 15 percent of its calories from fat, 70–80 percent from complex carbohydrates, and 10–15 percent from proteins.

In each of the 4 stages, your child can eat unlimited quantities of vegetables, fruit, whole grains, legumes, and, if you choose to include them, nonfat milk and yogurt and egg whites. Nuts may be eaten in moderation as the once-a-day snack during Stage 1 but should be avoided in Stages 2, 3, and 4, because of their very high fat content. Chestnuts are a low-fat exception.

Vegetables Best

Of the Stage 4 foods, vegetables are more nutritious than fruit when, calorie for calorie, their nutrients (vitamins, minerals, protein, and fiber) are compared. Below are actually two lists. On the left are vegetables and fruits arranged in decreasing order of their nutritional contents, often called nutritional density. The other list, on the right, is arranged in decreasing order of consumption by Americans.

18 of the Best Stage 4 Foods

Nutritional Density		Order Consumed
Broccoli	1	Tomatoes
Spinach	2	Oranges
Brussels sprouts	3	Potatoes
Lima beans	4	Lettuce
Peas	5	Sweet corn
Asparagus	6	Bananas
Artichokes	7	Carrots
Cauliflower	8	Cabbage
Sweet potatoes	9	Onions
Carrots	10	Sweet potatoes
Sweet corn	11	Peas
Potatoes	12	Spinach
Cabbage	13	Broccoli
Tomatoes	14	Lima Beans
Bananas	15	Asparagus
Lettuce	16	Cauliflower
Onions	17	Brussels sprouts
Oranges	18	Artichokes

It's obvious from the above lists that Americans are not eating the most nutritious choices.

Fiber

The Stage 4 diet is very high in fiber, supplying 25–30 grams per day for teenagers and 10–15 grams for younger children—the amount of daily fiber recommended by the National Cancer Institute, and about three times the amount in the typical Western diet. The fiber is of two types. Soluble fiber, from a variety of grains and legumes such as oat bran and beans, has the effect of reducing blood-cholesterol levels. Insoluble fiber, contained in many vegetables and wheat bran, moves digested food through the intestines more quickly. This type of fiber is thought to prevent cancer of the colon. Many people are not aware that neither meat nor dairy products—nor any other animal product—contains fiber.

Animal products have no fiber at all. None!

As your child moves through Stages 1, 2, and 3, the soluble and insoluble fiber in her diet will increase to the ideal level. While she consumes this much fiber, water intake is important, to keep the fiber spongy and moving through the bowel. At least six to eight 6-ounce glasses of water daily are needed on the Stage 4 diet. Water is the primary "beverage" for Stages 1, 2, 3, and 4. Anything else is considered a snack.

Nonvitamin and Nonmineral Ingredients

As already discussed, vegetables and fruits contain hundreds, maybe thousands, of substances that are not vitamins or minerals, and have no nutritional qualities, but appear to offer a protection against cancer. These are the phytochemicals—not found in any vitamin or mineral supplement—which are plentiful in the Stage 4 diet. In fact, this is practically the *only* place they are found. For example, broccoli contains the phytochemicals *isothiocyanate* and *indoles;* citrus fruits, *limonene;* tomatoes, *p-coumaric acid* and *chlorogenic acid;* onions, *allyl sulfides;* dried beans, *phytosterols;* and grains are rich in *phytic acid*—and all have cancer-inhibiting or preventing properties. It is probable that thousands more exist that haven't been discovered. This explains why study after study has shown far less cancer among people eating an abundance of vegetables and fruit. An-apple-a-day, loaded with *flavonoids,* was good advice.

The Potassium-Sodium Ratio

Generally, for good health it is considered best to consume far more potassium than sodium, approximately four times as much. The National Academy of Sciences estimates the daily *minimum* requirement of potassium to be 1,400 mg at age 2 and 2,000 mg at age 18. A diet of fruits and vegetables provides the proper ratio of potassium to sodium, but·the reverse is true of the typical American diet of meat, milk, and oils. You need not be concerned about this for your child on my Stage 4 diet, which supplies far more potassium than sodium.

Excess sodium is related to hypertension in some, but not all, children and adults. Only 15 percent of the sodium consumed comes from the salt shaker; the remaining is from processed and canned foods and baked goods or added during cooking. According to the National Academy of Sciences, the daily requirement of sodium for children between the ages of 2 and 18 is a *minimum* of 300–500 mg per day. This amount of sodium, also meeting the approval of the AAP's Nutrition Committee, is easily consumed by eating only vegetables, fruits, grains, and legumes. A reasonable upper limit of 1,800 mg per day would allow children to use ketchup, mustard, and some salt from the shaker on vegetables. In my experience, it takes very little salt on the surface of vegetables to make them far more palatable to most children.

I've called Stage 4 the "gold-standard" diet in my seminars, because it has every feature known to prevent the chronic diseases I have already discussed. It's very low in total fat, saturated fat, and cholesterol, and very high in fiber. Approximately 70 percent of its calories come from complex carbohydrates. It is the perfect diet, against which all others must be measured.

Once your child has remained on the Stage 4 diet for 3 to 12 weeks, she will prefer it to the fat-laden food from animal sources. Her "fat taste" will have disappeared—and if she stops eating these unhealthy foods, the "fat taste" will never return.

Chapter 14

A Low-Fat
Shopping Primer

A supermarket shopper for low-fat foods, like almost everyone else, relies on packaged, often processed, convenience foods—it's a fact that fewer people are cooking "from scratch." A 1993 survey showed that, of the nearly 30,000 items in the average supermarket, convenience foods and low-fat "guilt-free" foods and "healthy" snacks accounted for the largest recent sales growth. During the prior year, of the 12,312 new items introduced, one-fourth were promoted as being "low-fat."

Go In and Turn Right

The low-fat shopper should start in the produce department, on the far right as one enters our hypothetical food market. Here almost *everything* is a complex carbohydrate, low in fat and cholesterol, and high in fiber. You can scarcely go wrong, with two exceptions: coconuts and avocados. Coconuts are very high in the dreaded saturated fat, and avocados contain excessive saturated and monounsaturated fat. It's best to avoid both.

As discussed in Chapter 9, the fruits and vegetables found in the produce department are available in an astonishing number of varieties. Those with the most intense color are usually the most nutritious. For example, approximately 1 cup of spinach supplies the daily requirement of all vitamins, whereas 27 cups of iceberg lettuce are required to supply the same vitamins.

Produce departments are stocking many of the new hybrid fruits and vegetables described in Chapter 9. In 1992 alone, 50 were introduced to the market. Many of these are just variations in size and color, offering no added nutritional value, but there are exceptions. Sweet-tasting "broccoflower" has double the vitamin C and folic acid of either of its parent vegetables, broccoli and cauliflower. A white tomato contains less acid. Beta carotene is three times as plentiful in a new carrot called Cara-Bunch. These hybrids are more expensive, and their added nutrients are probably not worth the money, according to New York University's top nutritionist, Marion Nestle. "This isn't about good eating," Nestle said in a *U.S. News & World Report* interview; "it's about selling more food and growing it cheaper." There are exceptions: a new cucumber called Fanfare is a favorite because of its taste, size (about 9 inches), and resistance to disease. Genetically engineered vegetables will add to these varieties (see page 81).

Buy fresh vegetables and fruits whenever possible. The next-best choice would be the frozen product, since canned foods often contain excessive sodium or preservatives. As always, label reading is important here; even frozen vegetables and fruit may contain salt or preservatives. Otherwise, frozen and canned products are nutritionally equivalent to the fresh variety. The differences are marginal. When canned vegetables must be used, rinse them in plain water to remove the salt.

The next-most-important part of low-fat shopping is for grains and foods made from them. Moving to the aisles to your left in our store, stop when you see the long aisle of cereals. This aisle is confusing—all those boxes with their health claims. Here you should look for less sugar, more fiber, and less fat, all three of which should be on the label. Sugar may be listed here as a *simple* carbohydrate—as opposed to a complex carbohydrate. Stick with the less refined cereals, such as oatmeal, oat bran, rye, shredded wheat, Grape-Nuts, and the puffed-grain cereals such as Puffed Rice and Puffed Wheat. The best cereal choices should contain no fat,

3 grams or less of sugar, and at least 3 grams of fiber per serving.

Move on down the aisles and stop when you see the breads. Most are rich in complex carbohydrates, low in fat, and high in fiber, especially whole-wheat, sourdough, and French—but avoid croissants, doughnuts, cakes, and pastries. Plain, whole-wheat, and onion bagels and English muffins are excellent low-fat snacks. Angel-food cake is fat-free, and its sugar (a simple carbohydrate) is not harmful when limited to one serving a day in Stages 1, 2, 3, or 4. Rice and pasta should be in your shopping cart before you move on.

Brown rice, with its bran intact, contains a bit more fiber, folic acid, iron, riboflavin, and potassium than white rice, with the bran removed. Many people are surprised to learn how little difference there actually is between enriched white rice and brown rice. Both contain, per ½-cup serving, 115 calories and zero fat; fiber, 1 gram in white versus 1.5 grams in brown; niacin, 1 mg versus 1.4 mg; riboflavin, 0.01 mg versus 0.02 mg; thiamin, 0.12 mg versus 0.1 mg; and iron, 0.9 mg versus 0.5 mg. Their protein content is identical (3 grams). Therefore, you may buy and eat fortified white rice, the commonly found supermarket variety, totally gult-free, but keep in mind that brown rice may contain nonvitamin, as-yet-undiscovered healthful ingredients. Long, medium, and short grains clump together differently when cooked; most Western consumers prefer the long-grain (fluffy) variety, and Asians, using chopsticks, prefer a short-grain rice. All three are available in both brown and white forms.

All types of pasta are made from finely ground grain (flour) and water. Complex carbohydrates supply 82 percent of their calories; the rest is protein. A 1-cup serving of pasta made from refined, enriched wheat flour is fat-free and sodium-free, offers good levels of B vitamins and iron, and contains the same amount of protein as 1 egg. The big difference between refined-wheat pasta and whole-wheat pasta is the fiber content. The pasta "cut"—angel hair, spaghetti, or fettucini, e.g.—is nutritionally unimportant. A 3.5-ounce serving of whole-wheat pasta contains 5 grains of fiber (compared with 1.6 grams in regular pasta).

Beans and Peas

Legumes, commonly called beans or peas, will be found somewhere near the middle of our store. Beans are a necessary part of the Stage 3 and 4 diets. They are loaded with both soluble and insoluble fiber, low in fat, cholesterol-free, the best source of protein among all plants, and rich in vitamins and minerals.

Legumes are also versatile and inexpensive. You may serve them as an entrée or add them to spaghetti sauces and salads. They may be bought fresh, canned, or frozen. Like all canned foods, canned beans are usually high in sodium and should be rinsed. Some canned beans may be high in fat, such as refried beans, so it's important to read the label. Frozen beans and peas are OK if you rinse away any added fat, salt, or preservatives.

Canola, the Vegetable-Oil Champ

Vegetable oils must be chosen for the least amount of saturated fat possible, and the winner is canola oil, with only 6 percent saturated fat. In decreasing order of acceptance for the shopper, the other oils are: safflower oil, 9 percent; sunflower oil, 10 percent; corn oil, 13 percent; and olive oil, sesame oil, and soybean oil, each with 14 percent. The varying amounts of monounsaturated fat contained in these are not as important as their lack of saturated fat.

Just for comparison, you may want to look at the containers of lard, with 40 percent saturated fat; butter, 62 percent; and coconut oil, 87 percent saturated fat (commonly used to prepare popcorn). Get a small bottle of canola oil and a smaller bottle of olive oil. For Stages 3 and 4, you will need a can of spray-on Pam.

While you are comparing oils, think about nonstick cookware, if you don't already own some. It's possible, with the newer coatings (such as Excalibur or Du Pont Silverstone), to sauté and "fry" foods without butter and oils. According to the Food and Drug Administration, these may be scraped with metal spoons and spatulas without worry. Your supermarket may sell these; if not, it's worth a trip elsewhere. But you should be prepared to pay up to four times the standard cookware price for these heavier pans with extra-hard coatings. Most are stainless steel with aluminum or copper cores. According to a March 9, 1994, *New York Times* report, a Farberware Millennium 12-inch omelette pan costs $85.00, and a Magnalite deep 12-inch sauté pan $148.00. Both have Excalibur, the most common coating on nonstick pans, which is a stainless-steel alloy made by the Whitford Corporation that is integrated with the pan itself.

Snacks

Nearby will be the snack-food aisle, a nutritional mine field. You'll find that low-fat and nonfat cookies abound. As already discussed, even the low-fat and fat-free varieties are relatively high in calories because of their concentrated-fruit base.

Reduced-fat varieties of very high-fat snacks are generally to be avoided. Many contain between 20 and 40 percent less fat than the original products, but this is still too much fat. Jayne Hurley, nutritionist for the Center for Science in the Public Interest, commented in an Associated Press interview: "Reduced-fat versions of fatty foods don't make them healthy."

The leader (no contest) in true nonfat snacks, both with and without this excess of calories, is Nabisco. Examples of some of their relatively low-calorie nonfat products are SnackWell's Wheat Crackers, SnackWell's Cracked Pepper Crackers, and Mr. Phipps Pretzel Chips; all are fat-free with only 50–60 calories per serving (5 to 8 crackers or chips). Their per serving sodium content is 160 mg, about 10 percent of the daily allotment in a child's healthy diet.

As a rule, stay away from anything that ends in "-tos," like Doritos and Fritos, which are loaded with fat. For example, Crunchy Cheetos contain 12 grams of fat in a 1¾-ounce serving. These snacks are very difficult to overlook on the shelf, since Frito-Lay, a division of PepsiCo, completely dominates the potato-chip and tortilla-chip market. Data collected by Information Resources' InfoScan service from U.S. supermarkets, drugstores, and mass merchandisers for 1993 showed Frito-Lay with a 41-percent share of the $2.1-billion potato-chip business.

An 8-ounce bag of regular potato chips contains nearly 6 table-spoons of oil and supplies up to 80 grams of fat, according to the *University of California at Berkeley Wellness Letter*. This is nearly double your child's allotted fat for a day. It isn't easy to find a package of potato chips with less than 6 grams of fat per 1-ounce serving—this means at least 50 percent of calories from fat, usually much more—that doesn't taste like cardboard. Taste tests by the *Nutrition Action Healthletter* (November 1993) of 4 brands with less than 1 gram of fat per serving chose Louise's Fat-Free and FitFoods Fat-Free as the winners. Popsters, from American Grains, has passed the taste test among my patients. There are many selec-tions of pretzels that are totally fat-free; the best selections are those with very little salt. A 1-ounce serving of Barbara's Mini Whole Wheat Pretzels contain only 10 mg of sodium. Salt may be rubbed or scraped off regular pretzels without difficulty.

This completes the shopping tour for the Stage 4 ideal diet. While your child is at Stages 1, 2, and 3, however, you will have to visit the meat and dairy departments.

Meat and Dairy

The meat counter is where you will find the biggest source of fat for the family diet, so look for the leanest cuts to use while in Stages 1 and 2 of your child's—and, we hope, the entire family's—new diet plan.

The white meat of skinless chicken and turkey, along with finfish and shellfish, represents the lowest fat content. *Avoid duck and goose, which may be higher in fat than red meat*. Beef is a giant step up the fat ladder. Prime beef is highest; choice and select beef are somewhat less fatty.

When buying any meat, plan on serving 4 ounces of uncooked (3 ounces of cooked) meat per child per day while in Stage 1 (or three times a week while in Stage 2). The cooked servings may be 4 ounces for yourself and other adults. Buy it with very little visible fat, because you are going to have to trim the fat off.

Some processed beef and poultry are labeled to be a certain percentage fat-free. Keep in mind that this is based on *weight* and shouldn't be confused with percentage of calories from fat, which is used in all nutritional guidelines. For example, a package of meat may be 95-percent fat-free by weight, but derive more than 40 percent of its calories from fat.

The white meat of poultry contains less fat than dark meat, with skinless white meat the least fatty of all. The skin of chicken and turkey must be removed *before* cooking. Otherwise, much of the fat enters the meat. Beware of ground chicken or turkey, since the skin is usually included.

Remember that, among finfish, warm-water varieties, like flounder and snapper, are lower in fat than cold-water fish, such as salmon and mackerel. Shellfish, such as scallops, shrimp, and lobster, contain as much cholesterol as many cuts of beef but are *very* low in saturated fat, which makes them good selections for Stages 1 and 2.

All poultry and fish, even though low in fat, contain approximately the same amount of animal protein as equal servings of beef. This, and the fact that their fiber content is zero, disqualifies them for the Stage 4 diet.

Meat Choices for Stages 1, 2, and 3

	Calories	Fat (grams)	Saturated fat (grams)
Choice top sirloin, lean, fat trimmed, broiled, 3 oz.	170	6.6	2.6
Choice top round, lean, fat trimmed, broiled, 3 oz.	160	5.0	1.7

Meat Choices for Stages 1, 2, and 3 *(cont.)*

	Calories	Fat (grams)	Saturated fat (grams)
Chicken breast with skin, roasted, 3 oz.	167	6.6	1.9
Chicken breast without skin, roasted, 3 oz.	142	3.1	0.9
Salmon, Atlantic, cooked dry heat, 3 oz.	155	6.9	1.1
Snapper, Cooked dry heat, 3 oz.	109	1.5	0.3
Shrimp, grilled or baked, 3 oz.	86	1.3	0.3

Meat Substitutes

Meatless burgers and franks are available in most supermarkets. These, along with meatless Canadian bacon, chicken fillet, ground beef, and even sausage, are available with a reasonably low-fat content. Made from soybeans, these are good sources of vegetable proteins in a form your child will probably appreciate. The soy meat substitutes, although they contain much less fat than beef, are not fat-free. Nonsoy, fat-free vegetable meat substitutes are available from Wholesome and Hearty Foods, Inc., and are sold at large supermarkets. Their Garden-Veggie is made of mushrooms, brown rice, onions, nondairy cheese, rolled oats, broccoli, carrot, bulgur wheat, squash, red pepper, and garlic. Similar ingredients are found in their Garden-Sausage and Garden-Mexi. All three products contain about 7 percent of the daily sodium limits per serving. My reports from children: "Excellent taste!"

The fat-free varieties are fine for the Stage 4 diet. Label reading is advised, however, since some meat substitutes are relatively high in fat and sodium. For example, Heartline Imitation Canadian Bacon contains 7 grams of fat per serving, whereas the same brand's "lite" version is totally fat-free. The fat, from soybeans, is mostly unsaturated.

Most vegetarian "burgers" sold in supermarkets are not fat-free, containing approximately 6 grams of fat. However, fat-free "ground beef" is also sold by Heartline. Many other brands of totally fat-free meat substitutes are found in health-food stores.

Brush by the Dairy Shelves

While at the back of the store, you may want to pick up low-fat (1-percent) milk for the Stage 1 phase of your child's diet. For Stages 2, 3, and 4, if any dairy products are consumed, they must be skim milk or fat-free dairy foods.

Nearby you will find eggs, which you may want to buy to use the whites. Fat-free egg substitutes, such as Egg Beaters and Omelette Mix, are found near the whole eggs.

Fat-free dairy products, egg whites, and fat-free egg substitutes are, like low-fat fish and seafood, still high in animal proteins. I would like your child, when he reaches Stage 4, to consume at least 90 percent of his proteins as the vegetable variety, because of the heart-disease and cancer risk posed by animal proteins and the potential allergies from milk protein.

On this shopping trip, if you are a family of four already in Stage 4, your shopping cart might now contain the following items: a variety of deeply colored fresh vegetables and fruit; two boxes of fat-free, sugarless cereal, containing at least 3 grams of fiber per feeding; two loaves of whole-wheat bread; one dozen plain, whole-wheat, or onion bagels; two packages of fat-free crackers; two cans of red beans; one bag of dried beans; two packages of brown rice; one package of whole-grain pasta; one can of fat-free tomato sauce; one dozen eggs or an egg substitute; two quarts of skim milk (optional); several varieties of fat-free meat substitutes; one spray can of Pam; one bottle of "no salt added" ketchup; one jar of plain mustard; and a fat-free salad dressing. As I have already discussed, if you don't have nonstick cookware with the new Excalibur or Silverstone coating, and if the supermarket doesn't have any, you may want to visit a discount or department store on your way home.

Now you are finished. See how much easier shopping becomes when you and your children are eating right!

---

10 Tips for Low-Fat Shopping

1. Spend most of your time in the produce department.
2. Try new varieties of vegetables and fruit. Look at those with the most intense colors.
3. Don't forget about pasta made from whole grains.
4. Go straight for the bread counter, not the bakery.
5. Buy unrefined, low-fat, sugarless, high-fiber cereals.
6. Don't underestimate nutritionally dense beans, whether dried, frozen, or canned.
7. When buying packaged or canned food, read labels.
8. Buy low- or no-fat snacks; there are many choices. Careful, some are high in calories.
9. Buy small, lean cuts of meat for your transition stages.
10. Skim milk and nonfat dairy products during Stages 2, 3, and 4, and low-fat (1-percent) milk and low-fat dairy products during Stage 1, are allowed but unnecessary.

---

6 Tips to Combat Health-Hype

1. "No Cholesterol" on the package doesn't mean "low-fat."
2. "Low-fat" doesn't always mean "low-calorie."
3. Fat-free percentage is expressed in terms of weight, not percentage of calories from fat.
4. Oat bran may be present in token amounts, and therefore the product may not lower cholesterol levels.
5. The word "natural" doesn't guarantee quality.
6. "Low-fat" (2-percent) milk derives 35 percent of its calories from fat.

One-Stop Shopping

All of the low-fat foods and ingredients I have discussed here are usually found in any large supermarket. It is not usually necessary to seek out alternate suppliers and health-food stores. In fact, many items formerly found only in health-food stores are now on the shelves of supermarkets. On the other hand, health-food stores have expanded their product lines during the past 2 decades, and the shopper who wants *additional* low-fat choices may wish to visit them for secondary shopping.

Updated Food Labels

Healthy, low-fat, high-fiber foods are shelved adjacent to their high-fat, low-fiber counterparts, so you'll need to read labels carefully. You'll find them on all packaged foods as of May 1994, thanks to new federal regulations.

Revised federal food labels were mandated by the Nutrition Labeling and Education Act of 1990. These labels, a boon to shoppers, show exact total-fat and saturated-fat content of servings of all frozen, packaged, and canned foods. Serving sizes are standardized, and foods must meet standards if claims are made about cholesterol, fat, fiber, sugar, or calories. Also, nutrients, including fat, saturated fat, cholesterol, sodium, carbohydrates, fiber, calcium, and vitamins A, C, and D must be listed as percentages of daily needs, expressed as % Daily Value. Unfortunately, hydrogenated fat is counted as *total* instead of saturated fat.

Manufacturers are not permitted to use the term "low-cholesterol" on a label unless the food is also low (no more than 2 grams per serving) in saturated fat. The term "cholesterol-free" requires that a serving contain no more than 2 mg; "low-cholesterol," no more than 20 mg; "fat-free," less than 0.5 grams; "low-fat," less than 3 grams; "sodium-free," less than 5 mg; "low-sodium," less than 140 mg; "calorie-free," less than 5 calories; and "low-calorie," 40 calories or less.

The terms "light" and "lite" can be used only under two conditions: For foods deriving 50 percent or more of their calories from fat, the fat content must be reduced by 50 percent or more per serving. Foods deriving less than 50 percent of their calories from fat may be called "light" or "lite" when the fat is reduced by at least one-third per serving. These terms may also be used to denote a light-colored food, but the label must make that understood. Milk, once again, gets special consideration due to pressure from the dairy industry. Two-percent milk may continue to be labeled as "low fat" even though 35 percent of its calories are from fat.

If a food contains more than 11.5 grams of total fat or 4 grams of saturated fat per serving, it may make *no health claims at all*. However, health claims may be made when fiber content per serving is at least 10 percent of recommended daily needs; the term "high-fiber" may be used for foods containing 20 percent or more of the daily fiber needs.

In a *Wall Street Journal* interview, FDA Commissioner David Kessler said that the new labels were "one of the most important public-health landmarks this agency has ever engaged in. Before I took this job I had no idea whether six grams of fat per serving was high, medium, or low. . . . . Now we'll have a pretty good idea what that means."

The labels still do not list the percentage of calories from fat per serving. You can do this quickly, however, with a mental calculation using the following formula:

$$\text{Percent of calories from fat} = \frac{\text{Grams of fat per serving} \times 9}{\text{Total calories per serving}} \times 100$$

For example, one serving of Nabisco Grahams (2 crackers) contains 1 gram of fat. One serving also supplies a total of 60 calories. Since each gram of fat produces 9 calories, the "fat calories" $(1 \times 9 = 9)$ are divided by the total calories per serving (60): $9 \div 60 = 0.15$. Multiply this by 100 to convert to percent of calories from fat.

Or, since the labels now show the *number* of calories per serving from fat, you may just divide this number by the number of total calories per serving to get the percent of calories from fat.

To become a better label-reader, write for the free booklet *How to Read the New Food Label* (distributed by the Consumer Information Center, Department 79, Pueblo, Colorado 81009), prepared by the AHA and the FDA.

Vegetables, Fruits, and Pesticides

When shopping for vegetables and fruits, the consumer may, understandably, harbor a concern about bacteria, fertilizers, and pesticides on the surface of the food. Fertilizer and bacteria are best avoided by insisting on clean, fresh produce. And, although I would prefer the least amounts of pesticides possible, their health risk, according to most authorities, is far outweighed by the enormous benefits of a diet rich in vegetables and fruit.

The Alar-treated apple scare in 1989 was an example of the public's worry about the safety of eating fresh fruit, but there was more to come. Newspapers reported in 1993 that the insecticide endosulfan, which had been approved by the government for widespread use on crops of fruits and vegetables, may cause breast cancer. The suggestion was made because endosulfan and other insecticides may raise estrogen levels. Since there has been some evidence that estrogen may be related to breast cancer, someone recklessly suggested yet another cancer risk. No evidence existed that the insecticides were related to cancer in humans, but the pesticide scare was again enhanced, and parents continue to question the safety of fruits and vegetables.

Renewed concern among parents stems almost totally from what they have read or heard in the media. For example, the National Academy of Sciences (NAS), in its 1993 report *Pesticides in the Diets of Infants and Children,* concluded that there was "potential for concern." This was about all that most parents remember after reading newspaper accounts of the report.

The academy said that there was reason to suspect that, pound for pound, children may eat a lot more pesticides than adults. Kids eat more food for their size, and get less variety—sometimes eating nothing but bananas for a week straight, for example. The government, they said, sets pesticide-residue limits by looking at *adult* eating patterns.

This frightened both parents and health authorities, and *may unfortunately lead to a reduction of vegetables and fruit* in children's diets. A look at ongoing activities of the two federal regulatory agencies may be reassuring.

Pesticide Risk Exaggerated

In 1988, the Environmental Protection Agency took 86,000 samples of food and found that 81 percent had *no* detectable pesticide residues. More than half of these samples were of fruits and vegetables. Continuing annual inspections have shown the pesticide levels of fruits and vegetables to be far below the maximum safe levels established by the agency.

The Food and Drug Administration does a "market-basket" survey every two months. It analyzes pesticide residues in 117 kinds of food in five areas of the country, and has found the pesticide levels to be—with a few exceptions when the food must be with-drawn from the market—within safe levels. Its criteria for safe levels are based on standard animal-toxicity tests. Imported fruits and vegetables must meet the same safety requirements.

The World Health Organization and the Food and Agriculture Organization, agencies of the United Nations, have estimated that pesticides found on fruits and vegetables in the United States result in the ingestion of ¼ to 1 percent of the allowable amounts, even if consumed every day for a lifetime.

At least one large and prestigious private organization has looked into the pesticide risk of the national food supply. Jerry Taylor, director of natural resource studies at the Cato Institute, a privately funded Washington, D.C., "think tank" specializing in research and education on public policy, insists that our nation's food safety standards are adequate.

Greater chemical concentrations are found in milk, red meat, chicken, and turkey; fish contain both PCBs and DDT. Rachel Carson, in her pioneering book *Silent Spring,* eloquently described in 1962 how pesticides linger in fish and other animal tissues. Now, more than 30 years later, fish caught in Los Angeles County coastal waters contain high levels of DDT, which has not been manufactured since 1972. People who eat these coastal fish three times a week for three years are found to have five times the level of blood DDT as people who eat little or no fish. Vegetables and fruit can be washed and peeled, whereas the pesticides in fish, meat, and milk must be consumed along with the products.

Natural foods such as fat, animal proteins, and even excess calories, regardless of their source, may be a greater risk than pesticides. Dr. Ronald Hart, director of the National Center for Toxicological Research, has done extensive animal studies of diet-related cancer. He feels that the risk from pesticide residues on vegetables and fruits is small for children, compared to the known food-related risk of cancer from natural substances. Excess calories alone, he said, has been shown in his laboratory mice to be a cancer risk.

Children have been eating vegetables and fruit containing pesticide residues for almost 50 years, long enough for our epidemiological studies to have shown increases in cancer, birth defects, or neurological damage. This has not been found; on the other hand, diets *low* in vegetables and fruits are clearly associated with an increased risk of both cancer and heart disease.

According to former U.S. Surgeon General Everett Koop, children could have consumed the Alar in 16,000 apples without harm. He wrote in his memoirs, *Koop*, that during the past 40 years, while the use of pesticides was increasing, cancer of the stomach and rectum—the kind most likely to result from excessive pesticides—actually decreased by 75 percent and 65 percent respectively. The cancer rates that are increasing, he wrote, are cigarette-induced lung cancer in women and sun-induced skin cancer. He offered more reassuring facts: "The average American consumes 45 micrograms of *possibly* carcinogenic man-made pesticide residues every day. But that is practically nothing compared with the 500 micrograms of naturally occurring carcinogens in one cup of coffee, or the 185 micrograms of natural carcinogens in one slice of bread." Dr. Koop correctly points out that banishing all pesticides would leave us with rotting food and overgrowths of natural molds such as aflatoxin, which can be lethal.

Dr. Gladys Block, with the National Cancer Institute, made the reassuring statement to newspaper reporters: "I'm completely certain that the number of people who die as a result of eating pesticides on foods is vanishingly small, while the number of people who die becuse they haven't eaten enough fruits and vegetables is very large." Later, from her new post in the Department of Public Health at the University of California at Berkeley, she assured me that this opinion included any cancer risk for children. Another Berkeley scientist, Dr. Bruce Ames, director of the National Institute of Environmental Health Sciences Center, told *The New York Times* health editor Jane Brody in a July 5, 1994, interview, "I think pesticides lower the cancer rate." He considers pesticides an anticancer weapon because their use increases the yield of fruits and vegetables and lowers their cost, enabling more people to consume foods that appear to protect against cancer. As for animal studies, he said,

"Nearly half of all natural chemicals tested, like half of synthetic chemicals, are carcinogenic in rodents when given at high doses."

This conclusion was shared by many other scientists, including some on the National Academy of Sciences committee that issued the pesticide scare that frightened so many parents. Richard J. Jackson commented in a 1993 interview, "Given all the problems parents face in raising children, the added risk of pesticides in food is so small that it's not worth worrying about."

Like most consumers, I would prefer pesticide-free vegetables and fruit, but certified organic food is not currently produced in sufficient quantities and at affordable enough prices to feed all children. So what is the answer for those parents who are still sincerely concerned about the pesticide risk for their children, however small it may be?

It has been suggested by David Pimentel of Cornell University, in the university's *Handbook of Pest Management in Agriculture,* that pesticides could be *reduced* by 50 percent with no effect on crop yields or prices. Parents may seek out food that has been tested by independent companies, such as NutriClean, an Oakland, California, testing facility. NutriClean inspects more than 400 growers and provides weekly pesticide-residue testing of produce for more than 1,000 grocery stores nationwide. They have taken the position of an independent auditor, like a "Good Housekeeping Seal of Approval" for safe food. Also, locally grown vegetables and fruit, usually found at farmers' markets, are less likely to have been treated with pesticides and fumigants after harvesting.

How to Clean Fruits and Vegetables

Pesticide residues can be effectively reduced by peeling the fruits if you don't plan to eat the skin. For everything else, washing seems to be effective.

All produce should be washed with water and vinegar or a weak citric-acid solution to remove dirt and any surface pesticides, then rinsed thoroughly. A vegetable scrub brush should be used when cleaning items whose skin you will eat. You may chop spinach, broccoli, cauliflower, or other items that do not have smooth surfaces, before washing them. The outer leaves of cabbage and lettuce should be discarded, and the leaves and tops of celery should be trimmed.

Chapter 15

Back Home,
Getting Started

*S*ooner or later, you'll find yourself back home with a pretty good idea of what your child should be eating to prevent the chronic illnesses of later life. You may want to keep this book nearby for reference and place bookmarks at the beginning of Chapters 13, 15, 21, and 22. You will probably refer to these parts repeatedly.

You may want to photocopy pages 129–30, which outline the beginning and final goals of the programs through all 4 stages, for posting on your refrigerator or kitchen-cabinet door.

The first, "Dr. Attwood's Low-Fat Guidelines," consists of three columns. The left-hand column lists the things I want your child to discontinue eating right away. These are the problem foods that are unsuitable from the beginning of Stage 1. Soon they won't be missed. The middle column contains foods that may be eaten during the next few months, while in Stages 1, 2, and 3, in decreasing amounts. Some of these will not be eaten again when Stage 4 is reached. They too will soon be forgotten. The column on the right contains foods that will be eaten even after reaching Stage 4. I've kept these single-page charts very simple and basic; look back at Chapter 9 for detailed listings of the large variety of foods available for those on a Stage 4 diet.

Dr. Attwood's Low-Fat Guidelines

Discontinue on entering Stage 1	*Stages 1, 2, and 3 (plus any foods in Stage 4)*	*Stage 4— Any variety of:*
Whole milk, 2% milk, ice cream, butter, lard, and hydrogenated oils.	1% milk, low-fat yogurt, eggs.	Skim milk, nonfat dairy foods, egg white.
Untrimmed red meat, chicken and turkey with skin, duck and goose, sausage, bacon, cold cuts.	Vegetables, fruits, pasta, rice, low-fat or fat-free cereals, bread, beans, and peas.	Vegetables, fruits, pasta, rice, fat-free cereals, bread, beans, and peas.
All foods fried in oil. Cream and butter sauces.	Trimmed red meat, skinless chicken, turkey, and fish.	Nonsoy fat-free meat substitutes
More than 1 dessert and 1 snack daily.	One low-fat or fat-free dessert and snack daily.	One fat-free dessert and snack daily.

Vitamin B12 sources or supplements are recommended while in Stage 4 (see page 76).

Here is a further breakdown of the foods in each of the 4 stages:

4 Stages to an Ideal Diet

STAGE 1

- Limit meat, including poultry and fish, to 3 ounces (cooked) per day.
- Low-fat (1%) milk and low-fat dairy products if desired.
- No foods fried in oil.
- One dessert and 1 snack daily.
- Unlimited vegetables, fruits, grains, and legumes.

STAGE 2

- Limit trimmed meat, including skinless poultry and fish, to 3 ounces (cooked) no more than 3 times per week.
- Skim milk and nonfat dairy foods, if desired.
- No foods fried in oil.
- One low-fat dessert and 1 low-fat snack daily.
- Unlimited vegetables, fruits, grains, and legumes.

STAGE 3

- Trimmed meat, including skinless poultry and fish, no more than 3 ounces (cooked) once a week, or used sparingly as a condiment to vegetable dishes.
- Nonsoy fat-free meat substitutes.
- Skim milk and nonfat dairy foods, if desired.
- No foods fried in oil.
- One fat-free dessert and 1 fat-free snack daily.
- Unlimited vegetables, fruits, grains, and legumes.

STAGE 4

- No meat, poultry, or fish.
- Unlimited vegetables, fruits, grains, and legumes.
- Nonsoy fat-free meat substitutes.
- Skim milk and nonfat dairy foods, if desired.
- Egg whites, if desired.
- One fat-free dessert and 1 fat-free snack daily.
- Vitamin B12 sources or supplements.

"Quiet Cooking"

After choosing the kind of food your child will be eating and bringing it home from the supermarket, you must now consider the various ways low-fat food should be cooked. Obviously, frying is a thing of the past. The following cooking techniques will be the most useful: steaming, boiling, stewing, and baking.

These are examples of "quiet cooking," as opposed to the noisy frying that was once heard in your kitchen. In Robert James Waller's best-selling novel *The Bridges of Madison County,* Francesca Johnson, while making a vegetable stew for her new friend Robert Kincaid, realized that this was "quiet cooking."

> *After the pork chops and steaks and roasts she cooked for the family, this was quiet cooking. No violence involved anywhere down the food chain, except maybe for pulling up the vegetables. The stew cooked quietly and smelled quiet. It was quiet here in the kitchen.*

Other cooking methods you may use while your child is going through the 4 stages are roasting, stir-frying, grilling, broiling, and microwaving (see page 199 for more information on cooking techniques).

The "Family Plan"

Now you must decide what *you* will eat. When I give you my "Low-Fat Guidelines," and "4 Stages to an Ideal Diet," I strongly recommend that you and other members of the family adopt the same eating program. As adults, you already have some degree of coronary-artery and cancer risk from the diet you've been eating since childhood. Your benefits from this diet will be more immediate than those of your child, since you've almost certainly already developed some silent heart disease, which may be arrested or even reversed by the Stage 4 diet.

It becomes extremely awkward to shop for and serve your child Stage 4 foods if other members of the family are eating a typical high-fat diet. You wouldn't smoke in the presence of your teenager while asking him or her to avoid or give up the habit. Similarly, the fat taste, as I have discussed, is strongly influenced by social situations and, like smoking, is a habit that must be broken.

As mentioned, Victoria Moran has written an excellent essay for this book, "A Mom's Guide to Happy, Low-Fat Kids." This encouraging and helpful piece from a mother and health writer appears in Chapter 22. I regularly give it to the parents of my patients to take home. This guide alone, I feel, is worth the price of the book.

You'll find dozens of low-fat recipes in magazines and in the cookbooks listed under "Recommended Reading," in the back of this book. However, I wanted to give you something special, which you will not find in other cookbooks. Our unique "children-tested" recipes, developed exclusively for this book by 17-year-old Sonnet Pierce—whose avocation is low-fat cooking for her siblings and other children—can be found in Chapter 23.

I hope you will find all of the information contained in these sections both inspiring and useful.

Chapter 16

When Children Eat Out

*D*r. Peter Jones, of the Baylor University Lipid Clinic, advised a group of physicians at a conference, "If a restaurant has a drive-through window or delivers food to your home, don't eat their food!" He conceded, however, that some families, possibly including yours, will probably continue to eat in fast-food outlets and thus should learn what's best to eat there.

Avoid their standard burgers and French fries. Most fast-food restaurants now have salad bars; some offer baked potatoes, pasta, vegetables, and fruit. If a burger is a must for your child—while he is on a Stage 1 or 2 diet—stick to a plain beef burger, broiled if possible, and placed in a bun with lettuce and tomato. Mustard or ketchup should be used, not the restaurant's own sauces. This kind of burger contains about 10 grams of fat, including 4 grams of saturated fat. Not exactly low-fat, but better than a "standard" cheeseburger with mayonnaise, which contains 20 grams of fat, including 10 grams of saturated fat.

Meatless burgers are appearing at a few restaurants. An example is the Garden-Veggie, served under various names at such places as T.G.I. Friday's and Hard Rock Cafe. Its patty contains 190 calories, zero fat (unless cooked in oil), and an impressive 8 grams of fiber. The Gardenburger with cheese contains only 3 grams of fat. These estimates from the manufacturer are based on a 2.5-ounce patty; individual restaurants may serve larger portions. Not bad. The Center for Science in the Public Interest did a taste test and gave both a high score. These are the same products available in supermarkets from Wholesome and Hearty Foods decribed on page 117.

Half of All Meals
Are Eaten Away from Home

It is possible for your child to eat low-fat food almost anywhere, including the school cafeteria, fast-food outlets, family restaurants, fine restaurants, and even airplanes. Learning how to make the proper choice requires educating yourself and your child. This may become a major portion of his total nutrition, since the average child eats 198 meals away from home each year.

Almost *any* menu can be "altered" by a sympathetic chef; most are eager to please. They will usually gladly comply when asked to "sauté" with a little lemon and water, low-sodium soy sauce, or plain water rather than with butter. You may also ask that the sauces and dressings be served on the side. If your child is in the transition stages, 1, 2, or 3, and is therefore eating poultry, the chef should be asked to remove the skin *before* cooking.

Caution in Italian,
Chinese, and Mexican Restaurants

Pasta may be ordered without cream sauce, or with a tomato sauce instead, which is usually, but not always, low in fat. Some red sauces contain large amounts of oil, as discussed earlier, and they should be added to pasta in small amounts, using a fork instead of a spoon. In general, pasta dishes in Italian restaurants are safe only without the creamy sauces. The *Nutrition Action Healthletter* warned that if you order a 2.5-cup serving of fettuccini Alfredo you stuff your arteries with as much saturated fat as three pints of Breyer's butter-almond ice cream! *It contains 97 grams of fat, the equivalent of five McDonald's Quarter Pounders*. The newsletter called this dish "a heart attack on a plate."

In Chinese restaurants, you may choose relatively low-fat entrées such as Szechuan shrimp or stir-fried vegetables. These are the fat equivalents of spaghetti and red sauce. Cooking oils add significant amounts of fat to many Chinese dishes; egg rolls and all deep-fried items should be avoided. For example, a typical serving of Kung Pao chicken contains a whopping 76 grams of fat.

Nutrition Action Healthletter found that typical Mexican combination plates were also high in fat: taco salad with sour cream and guacamole contained 71 grams of fat; chiles rellenos, 36 grams; and beef and cheese nachos, 89 grams.

Dr. Michael DeBakey, writing in *Family Circle* magazine (February 22, 1994), suggests that when eating out, children and adults should choose foods cooked in tomato sauce, or baked, broiled, grilled (dry without added fat), poached, roasted, or steamed. Avoid foods described by such terms as "au gratin," "basted," "casserole," "creamed," "crispy," "fried," "in gravy," "with Hollandaise sauce," or "sautéed." Most sauces are high in fat, especially if they contain cheese or butter.

Fat sneaks into restaurant food in unexpected ways. Appetizers are often fried. Duck, as mentioned before, is as high in fat as most cuts of beef. The fat that is often added to otherwise low-fat entrées as butter, cream, sour cream, mayonnaise, or cooking oil can be replaced by lemon juice, mustard, and ketchup—essentially fat-free, and always available. Desserts are a mine field of fat, especially ice cream, chocolate mousse, cheesecake, and almost all pastries. Some low-fat desserts are mentioned on page 137.

Condiments Belong on Side Dishes

As discussed, once your child's chosen meal is served, you must stand guard to avoid added fat in the form of condiments such as salad dressings containing oil, butter, gravy, and sour cream. At the very least, insist that these items be placed in dishes on the side, so that they may be added in small amounts or not at all. Somehow waiters and waitresses have trouble hearing such instructions, so if there is any doubt, repeat the order while making eye contact; you must depend on the communication between the waiter and chef.

When such orders are ignored and food arrives at my table already smothered with high-fat condiments, I often send if back. Even the most nonassertive parent should insist upon this.

Almost any restaurant employs food servers capable of convincing the chef to get together a variety of steamed vegetables and a baked potato. This goes well with a dish of plain pasta with marinara sauce. Insist that sour cream, bacon bits, and other high-fat toppings for the baked potato be left off or replaced with fat-free yogurt and lemon juice. Salads can be topped with fat-free dressings—some others, such as blue-cheese, contain up to 32 grams of fat per quarter-cup—or lemon juice. I've successfully asked for such a meal at establishments ranging from my own casual neighborhood restaurant to onboard the *Queen Elizabeth 2*.

Salad bars are available almost everywhere, even in supermarkets and fast-food restaurants. They usually offer a variety of vegetables, fruit, and beans, but you shouldn't assume that everything found there is low-fat. Salad bars often provide high-fat salad dressings, fat-laden sauces, and even fried fish or chicken. As a general rule, when pieces of vegetables, fruit, and legumes can be seen individually without the camouflage of cheeses, creams, sauces, and dressings, they can be considered low-fat.

Among the low-fat salad-bar choices that I would recommend for your child are plain pasta salad, without meat or cheese, with a "lite" dressing; tossed salad of lettuce with cucumbers and tomatoes with a nonfat dressing; a variety of raw vegetables such as carrots, mushrooms, green peppers, and onions; cooked vegetables such as red beans and corn; and fruit.

The Hotel Breakfast Menu

Your child can eat from most hotel breakfast menus without resorting to high-fat food. English muffins are often on the menu. These and plain bagels may be ordered with jam or honey instead of butter or cream cheese. Eggs need not be purged from the traveling child's breakfast. Wonderful low-fat omelettes may be prepared by a knowledgeable chef by using two egg whites in place of each whole egg. Meat and cheese should be left out, but vege- tables, especially green peppers and onions, may be increased. Ask that the omelette be cooked with a very small amount of oil (one teaspoon or less) or a pan spray such as Pam. Most breakfast menus add hash-brown potatoes to an omelette dish, so tell them instead to serve your child whole-wheat toast without butter: children love making their own omelette sandwiches at the table. Here, ketchup, especially the low-sodium kind, goes well as a fat-free condiment.

Hot oatmeal is usually accepted by children if it is topped with lots of colorful fruit, such as strawberries, blueberries, bananas, or raisins, all usually available on hotel breakfast menus. Plain waffles with syrup, but not butter, are mistakenly thought by many parents to be a low-fat selection. Not so. A typical waffle, even without added butter, contains 11 grams of fat, including 2 grams of satu- rated fat.

Instant hot cereals, powdered skim milk, and fruit can be taken on trips to fill in when low-fat meals are unavailable. These may be taken into restaurants to supplement their limited low-fat menu. I've recommended this to the parents of my patients for many years. They say there's never any objection from a waiter or a waitress when they ask for a bowl, hot water, and a spoon.

Other low-fat restaurant choices for your child include soups made with clear broth (such as chicken noodle or vegetable), fruit salad, lean cuts of beef, poultry, finfish, and shellfish (while she is in Stages 1 and 2). A shrimp cocktail is practically fat-free. Some low-fat choices for desserts are frozen nonfat yogurt, angel-food cake, sorbet, gelatin, fat-free brownies, and fruit.

Airline Food

All major airlines will serve low-fat vegetarian meals for yourself and your child if you order them 24 hours before departure. Several, including American and Delta, will serve a vegetable meal, with or without dairy products, with a six-hour notice, so there is no excuse for eating the usually high-fat food served on most flights. If you have forgotten to arrange low-fat fare, there is almost no chance of finding something appropriate to eat on the plane. In that case, you can take along fat-free snacks, such as Fig Newtons, fat-free granola bars, bagels, or fruit in your carry-on bag.

As a final strategy for reducing fat while away from home, dietitian Hope Warshaw, author of *Eat Out, Eat Right,* suggests sharing portions with another person, placing "extra" food on a bread or salad plate, and asking the waiter for a "doggie bag"—not for you; for your dog, a carnivore.

Chapter 17

School Lunch Programs

In theory, school lunches are nutritionally
balanced meals; in fact, they are so
nutritionally poor that they're virtually
hazardous to a growing child's health.
                              —*Dr. Earl Mindell*
                         Parents' Nutrition Bible

*I*n 1993, 25 million children were regularly served school lunches,
at a cost to the federal government of $7 billion. Although the U.S.
Department of Agriculture (USDA) sets guidelines for operating
these programs, including that 30 percent or less of calories should
come from fat, there was no requirement that the individual school
districts must abide by these guidelines. They were free to buy beef
and dairy products and enter into contracts with food manufacturers
to make the finished product to be served to your child. Under this
arrangement, the food choices for most children may not be adequate to ensure a healthful diet.

Simply put, school lunches contain too much fat and too little of
carbohydrates and fiber. And if this is not bad enough, when I ask
students how the meals taste, their almost universal answer is
"Yuk!" My conclusion is based on my visits to school cafeterias,
talks with students and school food-service personnel, and analyses
of my patients' food diaries, which I encourage them to keep. A

USDA report made public on October 26, 1993, confirmed my observations (see below).

Children's Health "Deep Fried"?

Ellen Haas, assistant secretary for food and consumer services at the USDA, oversees the nation's school lunch program. In a *Newsweek* interview, she described a Baltimore school cafeteria: "The first thing you saw on the cafeteria line was french fries and pepperoni pizza. The second choice, french fries and a steak-and-cheese sandwich. The third choice was french fries and a fried-fish sandwich. The fourth choice was french fries and a submarine sandwich." Currently, schools get almost no fresh potatoes from the federal commodity program; rather, the fried variety are obtained from large food manufacturers.

The Baltimore school-cafeteria inspection was part of a national survey by the USDA. They inspected 545 schools during 1992 and found that 99 percent offered lunches exceeding the federal guidelines for total fat by 25 percent and saturated fat by 50 percent. Sodium recommendations were exceeded by 100 percent.

The survey showed that in the schools examined the average percentage of calories from fat was 38, and that the children were getting an artery-clogging 15 percent of their calories from saturated fat. There were deficiencies too. The children weren't getting enough fruits and vegetables. Carbohydrates supplied only 47 percent of calories, well below the USDA recommendation of 55 percent and my Stage 4 diet target of 70–80 percent. And, according to a *New York Times* report, at some schools the survey found that as little as 12 minutes was allowed for eating.

These findings prompted the USDA to hold regional hearings throughout the country concerning the nutritional quality of local school lunch programs. Even before the survey, critics of the nation's school lunch program had been compiling statistics. The Public Voice for Food and Health Policy, a consumer-advocacy group, announced in a press release, after the USDA report, that fewer than 10 percent of children ages 6 to 11 eat the USDA-recommended 5 servings a day of fruits and vegetables, and more than half eat less than a single serving of fruit a day.

Defensive after years of criticism by parents and knowledgeable health authorities, public-school food-service departments groped for a sensible response to the USDA report. The American School Food Service Association made no comment on the findings except to say that at least half of the school lunch programs in the country offer low-fat meals and that school lunches provide at least one-third of the daily requirements for vitamins A and C, calcium, and iron. They were apparently stung by USDA Secretary Mike Espy's public statement at a Washington, D.C., news conference: "We can't continue to deep fry our children's health." But individual school cafeterias were not required by federal law to comply with USDA recommendations.

Prior to the USDA's 1993 report, there was little indication that the federal government had taken a serious look at the excessive fat contained in school cafeterias. The NIH published guidelines for reducing saturated fat in school lunches in their *Child and Adolescent Trial for Cardiovascular Health (CATCH 1990)*. Under the heading "Tips to Reduce Saturated Fatty Acids in Food Preparation and Recipes for School Lunches," all 21 suggestions were concerned with alternate ways to serve meat, dairy products, and other high-fat foods. Nothing was said about limiting these foods and increasing servings of vegetables, fruit, whole grains, and legumes. Such guidelines are no great help to school food-service departments.

An Entire Generation Misinformed

How schoolchildren are taught to eat, according to Dr. Neal Barnard in his book, *Food for Life,* has remained essentially the same since 1956, when the Department of Agriculture introduced its 4 food goups. Two of these groups were meat and milk. So an entire generation thought these were the foundations of a healthy diet, and ignored their artery-clogging levels of saturated fat and cholesterol.

Today, the typical school lunch program continues to emphasize these 2 groups. Furthermore, as recently as 1994, schools were *required* by federal mandate to offer whole milk; the availability of low-fat and skim milk was left to the discretion of the individual schools.

Root-Beer Milk

The Western Dairyfarmers' Association plans to extend nationally a program successfully started in the Denver Public Schools to increase children's consumption of whole milk by making available an even higher-fat root-beer flavor. In an interview in March 1993, Denver's school food-services director, Donna Wittrock, wasn't worried about the extra fat. "They need the calcium, vitamins, and protein." She added that Denver's 23,000 public-school children are now consuming more whole milk, for the first time in years. "The benefits," she said, "far outweigh any drawbacks of a little more fat and sucrose." More heart attacks for the twenty-first century!

A few months later, a new national T-shirt design competition was won by Steven Barga, a 15-year-old from Staten Island, New York. The company sponsoring the competition, Designs for Education, had asked students to create interesting or provocative T-shirts that students could relate to. His winning design was a pie chart showing the fate of students consuming school lunches: "Fatalities, 70 percent; Food ate them, 10 percent; They ate food, 5 percent, and Survivors, 15 percent."

In her interview by the Associated Press on October 20, 1993, Donna Wittrock seemed to have taken the whole thing seriously enough to check scientific literature; she claimed to have found "absolutely no scientific proof for your statement about school food causing death for a student." The shirt design was intended to be a joke, but it appeared that food-service directors were getting edgy.

High-Fat Required, Low-Fat Optional

Parents hardly know what to expect when, during preschool or grade school, the child encounters foods prepared and served, for the first time, by strangers—so they simply trust that federal nutritional guidelines are required of the schools. Unfortunately, until 1995 the only requirements that had to be followed were those making available high-fat foods. They *must* have included specified servings (depending on grade level) of meat, milk, or other animal-protein sources.

These USDA requirements were intended to supply at least one-third of daily needs of each nutrient. Nothing in the design suggested that *reducing* animal fat was required. However, in keeping with the National Academy of Sciences' recommendation to reduce fat, some schools offered low-fat milk, usually 2-percent or skim milk. Often, this was the result of concerned parents who had banded together and pressed for the changes.

Another USDA program in all public schools where lunches are served is Nutritional Education and Training (NET). This is generally designed to promote, in the classroom, the healthful qualities of milk and meat, with little emphasis on the harmful effects of animal fats and protein.

By early 1994, the USDA, recognizing the shortcomings of the current laws, invited parents and others who were dissatisfied with the current state of school lunches in their communities to write to USDA/FNS/CND, 3101 Park Center Drive No. 1007, Alexandria, Virginia 22302. New legislation by Congress to give the USDA more power to enforce its nutritional recommendations was in the planning stages.

High-Fat Meals Save Money

The USDA commodity program for the nation's public schools has been nutritionally detrimental. Since the government buys surplus meat, poultry, butter, and cheese for distribution to schools, and pays a fixed higher price for the highest-fat products, this assures that the program will provide mostly high-fat commodities. Why would beef and dairy farmers produce a surplus of low-fat products when the USDA pays more money for more fat?

The USDA's intentions are good, but some of the manipulations by the individual school food-service programs are for one purpose only: saving money. A clerk in a large Southwestern state's agency for distributing the USDA's commodity program to its school districts revealed to me how her state's school lunch programs manipulate rules to save money at the expense of serving high-fat foods to the children. These schools are supplied commodities of meat, poultry, butter, cheese, flour, vegetable oil, and vegetables. They are also paid for each meal the school cafeteria serves.

The clerk said that most schools in her state use the commodities and cash in the following way: "Since the commodities are free, they send the meat and poultry to large food processors who prepare the final product into breaded nuggets and other high-fat servings. The most underused commodities are the fresh vegetables. The schools rarely ask for them." She said that individual schools instead serve french fries purchased from food suppliers.

The government's commodity program is only part of the problem, the clerk said. Education and training of the school food-service staff, as well as of the students and their parents, are necessary for significant change. Of course, the school lunch programs have captive consumers.

There is an enormous potential for schools to improve children's general nutrition. A New Orleans elementary-school survey done by the Louisiana State University Medical Center in 1992 revealed that approximately 93 percent of elementary students ate the food served by a school lunch program. In some areas, at last 50 percent of the students also ate breakfast at school. The study showed that the children consumed less than one-third of their daily calories from school lunches, but up to 80 percent exceeded the daily recommended (AHA) intake of fat and saturated fat.

School Lunch Success Stories

You may want to take action if your child's school lunch program falls short of your low-fat expectations. I have found that school principals and district superintendents have been receptive and open-minded when I've given them nutritional material for their food-service staffs. You can make a difference—talk to your principal about what you have learned from this book. Most of the programs described below started with a single parent or physician who recognized that he or she could do something locally to make a difference.

Bob Honson, director of nutrition for the Portland, Oregon, schools, started, in 1993, to introduce kiwi fruit, vegetable muffins, beef-barley stew, and spinach-romaine salad as an initial step in a plan to increase vegetable and fruit selections for the students. He found that participation in the school lunch plan was growing by the end of the year. Though it's hard to get people to change their habits, he said in a *Newsweek* interview, it can be done. Meanwhile, Honson added, "There hasn't been a single death from french-fry deprivation."

Increasing the number of lower-fat selections has been successful in other school districts as a means of reducing students' consumption of fat. Robert C. Whitaker, a pediatrician in Bellevue, Washington, reported in 1993 that students in 16 elementary schools in his community ate lunches containing an average of 36 percent of calories from fat. He thought that they ate this much fat for one reason: the schools were serving only high-fat foods, such as hamburgers, hot dogs, and pizza. He wondered if kids would eat leaner foods if they were disguised as familiar meals.

He had the school cooks offer a choice between high-fat burgers and fries, and slimmed-down versions of such old favorites as chili or spaghetti and meatballs, made with ground turkey instead of ground beef. The majority of the students chose the lower-fat selections about one-third of the time, and over eight months the fat content of the average lunch fell from 36 to 30 percent of calories, with no complaints from the children. His conclusion: modifying the foods kids already like can improve their diets.

Healthy children instinctively eat the correct amount and types of foods whenever a wide variety of choices is available. If, on a given day, all needed nutrients are not eaten, children will choose the ones they missed the following day. They can maintain optimal health by acquiring them over 48 or even 72 hours. This is a perfectly natural pattern of eating for the human species.

In my opinion, if Whitaker's school lunch modifications had also increased the variety of vegetables, fruits, and legumes—giving the children more options among these foods—the fat consumed would have almost certainly fallen even further. My patients generally agree: their preference is to be given a wider variety of choices and allowed to decide what to eat.

The LUNCHPOWER! Progam

The high fat content of most school lunches can be reduced by innovative education programs such as Minnesota's LUNCHPOWER! Intervention Program. This 1992 program by the University of Minnesota School of Public Health recruited a team of registered dietitians, food-service directors, and cook managers to reduce the fat and sodium content of school lunches. They did so by modifying recipes and food-preparation methods, and by identifying and selecting vendor products, such as cookies, that were lowest in fat. They also promoted nutrition education for students and parents during the five-month program.

In 34 elementary-school lunch programs, this team of professionals was able to reduce the grams of fat per student from 32 to 20, and to reduce the calories from fat from 40 to 28 percent.

A similar intervention in New Orleans, the ongoing Heart Smart study established by the Louisiana State University Medical Center, provided food choices in school lunches that reduced fat by 30 percent. A report of follow-up testing in 1992 indicated that the students who participated in the program showed greater health knowledge and lower cholesterol levels than nonparticipants.

A Model School Lunch Program

In 1988, a young child's mother wrote to Dr. Ted Diethrich, founder and medical director of the Arizona Heart Institute, asking for help. Her husband had died of a heart attack, and her grade-school child had a high cholesterol level. Her efforts to feed the child low-fat food were being undermined by the lunches served in the school cafeteria.

Dr. Diethrich enlisted the help of Jane L. Newmark, a registered dietitian with a master's degree in public-health nutrition and a national authority on the prevention of heart disease through nutrition. She developed the Arizona Heart Institute's *Heart Healthy Lessons for Children*, a nutrition-education program for elementary-school children.

At this time, it so happened that the public-school district in Chandler, Arizona, was already beginning to reduce the fat in its school lunches, so the program was enthusiastically adopted throughout the district. The teachers used the educational program in the classrooms, and the Chandler Schools Food Service reduced the fat content of food in the school cafeterias and the snacks served in the classrooms. The program included in-service training for the cafeteria staff on the relation of dietary fat to heart disease. Parents were involved in the educational program through open-house gatherings and monthly menu supplements explaining the program.

The Chandler experience began in 1989 and has been considered a great success by parents, school food-service personnel, and the children who have learned to make proper low-fat food choices both at school and at home.

The Arizona Heart Institute's *Heart Healthy Lessons for Children* has been adopted in schools in more than 20 states, in London, and in Canada at the time of this writing. Questions about food service in school cafeterias may be directed to Cathy Schuette or Jeanette Shipley, Chandler Schools Food Service, 1525 West Frye Road, Chandler, Arizona 85224, or call (602) 786-7000.

Health-Conscious Administrators

Roland Chevalier, superintendent of schools in St. Martin Parish, Louisiana, convinced his school board to set up a task force to study and establish a comprehensive health-and-wellness plan. The goal of the program, established in the fall of 1993, was to improve the nutritional standards for their school lunches by reducing fat, sodium, and cholesterol in the children's lunch choices. This included food served in the cafeteria and the school's vending machines, which now serve fruit juices and fruit instead of chips and carbonated drinks.

School administrators approved the establishment of one of the most unusual and progressive school lunch programs in the nation. At the Kimberton Waldorf School in Kimberton, Pennsylvania, children are served organically grown food, with a strong emphasis on vegetables, fruits, and whole grains. The school is located on a 400-acre farm, which includes a community-supported organic garden project. The program, directed by Andrea Huff, is designed to comply with the USDA recommendations of 30 percent or less of the calories derived from fat. "Lunch at the Waldorf," as the program is called by Ms. Huff, has been accepted with enthusiasm by students from kindergarten through twelfth grade since its inception in 1991.

The American Heart Association's Hearty School Lunch Program was established in 1992 to encourage healthful eating in the nation's school cafeterias. The program suggests no more than 30 percent of calories from fat, less than 10 percent of calories from saturated fat, and less than 300 milligrams of dietary cholesterol per day. School districts may obtain material by contacting AHA offices.

A formal plan based on the Hearty School Lunch Program and made available to Texas school districts is known as Health Star, Guidelines for Healthy School Meal Planning. This is available from the AHA Texas Affiliate, Inc., at any of their regional offices. The main office is located at 1615 Stemmons Freeway, Dallas, Texas 75207.

These AHA school recommendations are, in effect, based on the AHA Step I diet, an improvement over present school lunch programs, but not low enough to prevent coronary disease effectively. Parents, physicians, and dietitians wishing to urge the AHA's Hearty School Lunch Program to recommend further reductions of fat in its guidelines may call (800) AHA-USA1.

New School Lunch Legislation

As already mentioned, as of 1994, the USDA guidelines for fat consumption were not *required* to be followed by the schools they served, while a requirement *did* exist that meat or meat substitutes and whole milk be made available to every student. Meaningful changes will require new laws to "encourage" the USDA to enforce its own nutritional guidelines. Senator Patrick Leahy of Vermont, chairman of the Senate Agriculture Committee, introduced legislation (S. 1614) in 1994 to *require* school districts to comply with the USDA's low-fat dietary guidelines of no more than 30 percent of calories from fat and no more than 10 percent of calories from saturated fat, to increase dietary fiber, to reduce the consumption of sodium and sugars, and to increase the consumption of fruits and vegetables for all children served in school lunch programs by July 1, 1996. The Senate bill "Better Nutrition and Health for Children Act of 1994" requires the USDA to follow its own guidelines when buying commodities for school lunch programs. It makes available funding to help schools purchase additional servings of fruits, vegetables, and low-fat dairy products. The bill *eliminates the requirement that whole milk be served* and directs that the USDA purchase for schools additional amounts of low-fat cheese that will be in surplus after the whole-milk requirement is removed.

The act requires the USDA to make available, at the request of state agencies and schools, assistance and information about means for schools to obtain organically produced agricultural products including vegetables, legumes, cereals, and grain-based products—and assistance in offering increased choices of low-fat dairy products and lean meat and poultry products. Also, the bill requires state agencies to provide, through the Nutrition Education and Training (NET) programs, training aimed at improving the quality and acceptance of school meals.

And finally, the bill requires the USDA to assist elementary schools in drafting restrictions of the sale of competitive foods of minimal nutritional value, such as soft drinks and candy from vending machines, anywhere on elementary school grounds during lunch periods.

Strong support for the bill came from Hillary Rodham Clinton, the American Academy of Pediatrics, the American Cancer Society, the Food Research and Action Center, the Children's Defense Fund, Public Voice for Food and Health Policy, and the Center for Science in the Public Interest.

The full senate passed this bill in August 1994. Since a similar bill (H.R. 8) has been approved by the House of Representatives, this new legislation will probably be signed by President Clinton by the time you read this chapter. The USDA, as discussed earlier, is preparing for this first major step to improve children's nutrition since the National School Lunch Act and the Child Nutrition Act of 1966.

One thing is certain. Whatever happens to the nation's school lunch program, either through federal legislation or at individual schools by concerned parents' demands, could have an enormous impact on the nutritional status of children in America.

Part Three

So You
Want Proof?
The Scientific Basis

• • •

When a subject is highly controversial . . .
one cannot hope to tell the truth. One can
only show how one came to hold whatever
opinion one does hold. One can only give
one's audience the chance of drawing their
own conclusions as they observe the
limitations, the prejudices, the idiosyncrasies
of the speaker.

> —*Virginia Woolf*
> *(1882–1941)*

Chapter 18

The Childhood Beginnings
of Heart Disease

> As a cardiologist, I believe that many of
> the people I see in my office probably wouldn't
> be needing my help if they had learned the
> principles of low-fat living at an early age.
> —*Steven Van Camp, M.D.*
> *Director of Cardiac Rehabilitation*
> *Alvarado Hospital Medical Center*
> *San Diego, California*

*C*ardiologists are specially trained to treat and rehabilitate the adult victims of coronary heart disease, usually after the disease has progressed silently for several decades. Many, like Dr. Steven Van Camp of San Diego, have been convinced by a growing number of scientific reports that this disease begins at a shockingly early age. It is my intention, by reviewing these studies, to convince you beyond the slightest doubt that your child is already at risk.

I have asked you in Parts One and Two of this book to believe that excessive dietary fat leads to high blood cholesterol levels and the beginning changes that lead to coronary artery disease as early as the pre-kindergarten years; and that it progresses invisibly to its endpoint, usually in middle or old age, when symptoms finally appear in the form of sudden chest pain, a heart attack, or even sudden death. Preventing this scenario will undoubtedly be the new focus of pediatrics in the twenty-first century.

The scientific studies have, so far, been only briefly mentioned. Now I'll share with you more of the evidence that I've found so compelling. Many of these studies and surveys have been under way long enough to have followed preschool children well into adulthood. The most respected and longest ongoing investigation began in a small town in Louisiana more than 22 years ago.

The Bogalusa Heart Study

Findings of the Bogalusa Heart Study, reported in dozens of well-known medical journals, including the *American Journal of Cardiology* in 1992, seem to have been largely ignored by the medical profession. Dr. Gerald Berenson, then a professor of cardiology at the Louisiana State University Medical School, founded the study in 1973 to investigate the effects of diet and exercise on children in his hometown of Bogalusa, Louisiana. By 1994, its twenty-first year, more than 14,000 children had been followed by the program; the oldest had reached their mid-30s.

The study has shown that elevated cholesterol and LDL levels could be found in children as young as 6 months of age, and that those with high levels usually maintained them.

Most impressive were autopsy studies, beginning in 1978, of children in the study who had died suddenly of accidents and other causes of unexpected death. Fatty deposits—referred to by many pathologists as "fatty streaks"—were found in the aorta (the main artery leading out of the heart) of *all children* over the age of 3, and in the coronary arteries of most of the 190 children and young adults (between the ages of 3 and 33 years). Many of these children and young adults had been followed in the study for years, and *those with the highest known cholesterol levels had the most fatty deposits. This indicates a need to do something to control cholesterol levels during childhood.*

This evidence of the early-childhood beginnings of heart disease is not the first; signs of the disease were found in 3-year-old children in Europe as early as 1930. In 1958, Dr. R. L. Holman found these same fatty deposits in the aortas of *all* preschool children in a New Orleans study. More recent autopsy studies on children were done by Dr. H. C. Stary in 1989 and 1990. He found fatty deposits in the coronary arteries by age 3, and by age 12 nearly 70 percent of children examined had them. They increased in size rapidly throughout the teens; and virtully all young adults had the disease by age 21.

These findings, even though reported in major medical journals in America and Europe, remained of only academic interest. Practicing pediatricians and family physicians either paid no attention or were not made aware of the information. Even today, I rarely encounter a physician colleague or a doctor at one of my seminars who has ever heard of the studies by Holman or Stary, or even of the ongoing Bogalusa Heart Study, though it has been covered in 400 articles and 3 textbooks.

Dr. Basil Rifkind, director of the Lipid Metabolism–Atherogenesis Branch of the NIH's National Heart, Lung and Blood Institute— the agency that administers the National Cholesterol Education Program—wrote in an editorial that appeared in April 1993: "Aortic fatty streaks occur in individuals as young as 3 years old, and coronary fatty streaks occur in more than half of children aged 10 to 14 years. Approximately 8 percent of individuals aged 10 to 14 years have more advanced lesions." Dr. Rifkind went on to say that these deposits have been shown by the Pathobiological Determinants of Atherosclerosis in Youth (PDAY) Research Group to correlate with blood-cholesterol levels. This group's first report appeared in the *Journal of the American Medical Association* in 1990.

The PDAY Research Group that Dr. Rifkind was referring to, a large gathering of scientists and pathologists, in 1983 organized a multicenter cooperative project, involving nine university medical-research centers across the United States. Its mission was to study the natural progress of cholesterol lesions in children and young adults.

The group's latest report at the time of this writing *left little doubt about the early-childhood beginnings of coronary heart disease*. Among the 1,532 autopsies studied, aortic cholesterol lesions were found in *all* children between the ages of 15 and 19. Half of these already had lesions in the coronary arteries. Since such deposits are known to develop over many years, the group had—like the studies before it—once again proved the early-childhood beginnings of heart disease. They also concluded that it accelerates during the early teens.

The Johns Hopkins Young Adult Study

In a different study of slightly older young men, 1,017 medical students (average age 20) were followed for 42 years by Johns Hopkins researchers. Those with the highest cholesterol levels at age 20 were three times as likely to have heart attacks and nine times as likely to die of them. This 1993 report concluded that having high cholesterol at age 20 was one of the strongest predictors of later heart disease, even better than family history.

In older subjects yet, the Bogalusa Heart Study found cholesterol levels of moderate and high risk in 40 percent of 23-to-26-year-old men. Their autopsy studies found some degree of coronary disease in *90 percent* of *all* of these young adults. This was similar to the findings discussed elsewhere in my book, of young men of the same age range killed in battle during the Korean and Vietnam wars. "In the year 2030," said study director Dr. Gerald Berenson, "today's children with elevated cholesterol levels will become 1.5 million heart attacks and 500,000 needless deaths unless we change their eating habits now."

Which Children Are Already at Risk?

If we are to prevent this fate for yet another generation of children, it is first necessary to identify those who are already at high risk, which can only be done by checking every child's cholesterol level. As already discussed, the NIH, AHA, and AAP have decided against this. Their recommendation, based largely on a study of Iowa children, is for family physicians or pediatricians to check cholesterol levels of only those children whose parents or grandparents have a history of coronary-artery disease or a cholesterol problem. In my opinion, they have misinterpreted the findings of this important study.

Good Study. Wrong Conclusion.

The Muscatine, Iowa, study, reported in 1990 by the University of Iowa, has been quoted by the NIH and AAP as showing the "poor predictability" of children's cholesterol levels for elevated levels requiring intervention during adulthood. Both organizations used this study in formulating their guidelines for checking children's cholesterol levels.

The study followed the cholesterol levels of 2,367 children into adulthood. The NIH and AAP saw that, of the children with cholesterol levels in the highest 25 percent, only 25 percent of the girls and 44 percent of the boys had levels as adults high enough for dietary or drug interventions, according to NCEP guidelines. The study showed that, among children with cholesterol levels in the highest 10 percent, 43 percent of the girls and 70 percent of the boys had levels that would require intervention in adulthood. The NIH and AAP committees setting the guidelines for cholesterol screening in children apparently didn't feel that enough children maintained their high levels of cholesterol into adulthood to warrant checking *all* children's levels.

I reviewed this study very carefully and came to an entirely different conclusion. I thought the percentages of children with high cholesterol levels needing cholesterol attention as adults were quite high. Others have shared my opinion. It was a case of "Is the glass half full or half empty," agreed Dr. Berenson, when we talked at the 1st National Conference on the Elimination of Coronary Artery Disease in 1991.

Furthermore, it is likely that the adult levels of cholesterol considered to be high-risk, and needing intervention, will be revised downward soon, because of the recent studies showing that coronary disease *progresses* on a diet, recommended by the NIH, the

AHA, and the AAP, of up to 30 percent of calories from fat and 10 percent from saturated fat. The most notable of these studies were by Dr. B. G. Brown in 1989 and Dr. Dean Ornish in 1990.

Until 20 years ago, cholesterol levels up to 300 were accepted as tolerable by the medical profession. A level of 260 would have been satisfactory in the opinion of most doctors even 10 years ago. Then the satisfactory level was revised to 240, 220, and now 200, which is almost certainly still too high. As I have already discussed, the majority of heart attacks occur in people with cholesterol levels of 220 to 240.

Meanwhile, the NIH and AAP guidelines will miss *the one-third of America's children who are at risk and who may never know it until the disease strikes them later, as adults*. Under these guidelines, such children, without a family history of cholesterol problems or heart disease, will not have had a cholesterol-level check during their entire childhood.

I think this makes no sense. Is the cost of the test too great to justify identifying so many children who are at risk? The NIH and the AAP urge that *every* infant be tested for phenylketonuria, a rare genetic disease affecting only 1 child in 14,000; and every child is tested for lead poisoning to discover the 5 percent with high levels. The NIH also recommends hearing screening—at a cost of $300 per child—for *all* newborn infants to catch the 1 in 1,000 with deafness. According to estimates by the AHA, high cholesterol levels exist in 1 out of 3 children (40 million).

During a *Denver Post* interview, Dr. Berenson again expressed his disagreement with the NIH and AAP guidelines: "We screen children for hearing and vision, but they're not going to die from poor hearing or vision. They *are* going to die from heart disease. They are the next generation of heart attacks."

Check Every Child's Cholesterol

My position, published in 1992, in favor of universal cholesterol testing, is in direct opposition to the guidelines of the NIH, the AHA, the AAP, and even the AMA—notice how they agree on these purely arbitrary decisions. The "enormous expense" cited by these agencies—a cholesterol test on a child costs the physician about $2.50—must be compared with the cost of this disease, once it has developed—estimated at more than $100 billion annually in the United States.

Dr. Ronald E. Kleinman, then chairman of the Committee on Nutrition of the AAP, which set these guidelines for its member pediatricians, asked in a 1993 interview: "Why create an impression in a child that he or she is going to develop heart disease, when it may very well never happen?" I strongly disagree with his reasoning. According to the statistics made public by the National Center for Health Statistics—a division of the CDC—we can expect that half of all children living today will develop heart disease and one-third of them will die of it, just like their parents and grandparents.

Most Parents Are Young and Healthy

The NIH and AAP guidelines for checking children's cholesterol levels discussed above are based entirely upon whether or not a child's parents or grandparents have or have had coronary heart disease or high cholesterol levels. Using family history as a criterion for cholesterol screening in children is nonsense! As previously discussed, I contend that parents of most children are still too young to have manifested symptoms of coronary heart disease. Most parents have no idea what their own cholesterol level is.

And in many cases the family history is unknown. Data from a 1989 health census in Otsego County, New York, showed that, in 16 percent of the population, family health information was either unavailable or unknown for one of the parents.

Dr. Richard E. Garcia, codirector of the Pediatric Lipid Clinic at the Cleveland Clinic foundation, contacted 299 families of children with high cholesterol levels. Nearly half (48 percent) reported no history of high cholesterol or premature heart diseases in siblings, parents, grandparents, aunts, or uncles.

Another study shows us why we must know every child's cholesterol level. In a 1989 report by the Department of Pediatrics of Chicago's Northwestern University Medical School, family-history factors recommended by the NIH and the AAP as criteria for cholesterol screening in children did not identify half of all the children found to have abnormally high cholesterol levels. Among 1,005 children tested, 274 had cholesterol levels over 175. More than half of these had no family history of heart disease or elevated cholesterol levels. The study concluded that, in order to identify children with abnormally high cholesterol levels, *all* children must be tested at least once.

Pam Mycoskie, author of the best-seller *Butter Busters: The Cookbook*, confided in a newspaper interview that her brother had died of heart disease at the age of 19 though there was no known heart disease in the family. This resulted in her discovery of her own cholesterol level, which was 240. Obviously, it would have been advantageous if both had had cholesterol levels checked during childhood. In my practice, as previously mentioned, I have often discovered high cholesterol levels first in a child and later in his parent or older sibling.

Parents Want to Know

Can your child's cholesterol level be significantly lowered if you reduce the fat in his diet? Many pediatricians and nutritionists insist that this requires a level of compliance most parents or schools are not likely to get from children. Let me encourage you. In my clinic, I often first simply give the parent and child instructions on one sheet of paper (see page 129). The column on the far left lists the things children should discontinue eating at once. This includes whole milk, untrimmed meat, fried food, and oils. The column on the far right includes foods they can eat *more* of, and the middle column lists foods that need not be altered for the time being. This token diet intervention has usually resulted in a 10-percent drop in their cholesterol level within three weeks. Some children quickly learn to accept the challenge and are anxious to return for a cholesterol check.

The importance of identifying children with high cholesterol levels, regardless of their family history, will become even more obvious as you read the following descriptions of how dietary intervention can make a difference.

In 1991, the Mayo Clinic's Section of Pediatric Cardiology found that reducing the saturated fat in the diets of 32 children reduced their average cholesterol level in only three months. Though there were wide variations in how much each child's level decreased, the study concluded that it was practical to curb children's cholesterol levels over a relatively short period of time through diet. A significant correlation was found, for the group as a whole, between the drop in cholesterol levels and the change in grams of dietary saturated fat.

The Mayo experience was, of course, with a small group of children under dietary supervision for a short period of time. Larger groups of children in an uncontrolled environment such as schools have shown similar reductions in their cholesterol levels after both educational and dietary interventions.

In Chapter 1, I discussed the major difference between the cholesterol levels of boarding-school boys during the school term, while they were eating lower-fat selections, and their cholesterol levels at home during spring break and summer vacation, when they were on a higher-fat diet. This, the first of the diet-intervention studies on children, left little doubt that reducing a child's consumption of fat effectively reduced his cholesterol level.

Educational intervention alone has achieved similar results. The Know Your Body (KYB) Study, conducted by the American Health Foundation from 1979 to 1985, studied 1,105 children in the fourth grade. Approximately half (in eight schools) were given classroom instruction in diet, physical activity, and cigarette-smoking prevention, all related to coronary heart disease. Their parents received educational materials and attended seminar groups conducted by the study. The other half (students from seven schools) were not subjected to these classroom sessions. The program found, after five years, that the children who had received the educational intervention had lower cholesterol levels than the control group *and had a surprising 73-percent reduction in the rate of initiation of cigarette smoking.*

In another educational intervention, the researchers attempted to influence the whole family by teaching the children how to make low-fat selections. This program for 400 third- and fourth-grade children in Baltimore, coordinated by the Johns Hopkins University School of Medicine, concentrated on nutritional education. The children were taught to make better food choices in fast-food restaurants, at snack time, and in the grocery store. Three years later, the study showed, their cholesterol levels were much lower than at the start of the program. Dr. Kerry Stewart, who directed the program, said, "Kids don't die from heart disease; they die from it when they are adults." He said that his goal was to establish good eating habits now to prevent heart disease later. Another bonus found during the program, he said, was that kids taught their parents what they learned about reducing fat.

The Pawtucket Heart Health Program in Rhode Island works closely with 23 parochial and public schools. It's an educational program to teach junior-high-school students about the healthful effects of reducing their dietary fat. In 1988–89, 105 students participated in a "cook-off" program and were given scores for creative low-fat meals. At the beginning of the program, 40 percent of the students had elevated serum cholesterols (over 170 mg/dl). These children experienced a 10.7-percent drop in their cholesterol levels during the 12 weeks of the cook-off, during which (it was assumed by the investigators) the children became more aware of the harmful effects of fat in their diets.

The High-Fat Life-Style Is International

Most industrialized nations are experiencing high mortality rates from coronary heart disease. Dr. Ernest Wynder, president of the American Health Foundation, who had first warned his colleagues in 1952 of the relationship between smoking and lung cancer, has compared coronary deaths throughout the world with children's cholesterol levels. "Countries with the highest adult death rates from coronary artery disease," he told me, "also have the highest cholesterol levels in their children."

Since the diets of many countires are changing, especially in their urban areas, I started looking at the Asian studies, where I found that trends toward excessive consumption of fat among city children had been under way for several decades.

Trouble in Asia

No better model exists of the subsequent effects of children's dietary fat than that of the Japanese. Historically, they have raised their children on diets consisting of less than 10 percent of calories from fat. Accordingly, Japan is among the nations of the world with the lowest incidence of coronary disease in adults. Furthermore, life expectancy in Japan leads all other nations for which records are available. Unfortunately, as discussed, this sparkling example may not continue.

In the larger cities, the Japanese diet during childhood has become Westernized, with increasing levels of fat intake since World War II. Though the total number of calories consumed has not changed, daily fat intake was 16 grams in 1946, 27.8 grams in 1961, and 56.8 grams in 1985. Therefore, dietary fat has doubled during the last 25 years and nearly tripled during the postwar period. Between 1960 and 1991, a sharp drop in the consumption of grains was coupled with an increase in meat, whole milk, and oils. Low-fat dairy products are rarely consumed. A recent study in Japan, reported to *The New York Times* on April 13, 1994, by Dr. Teruo Omae, president of the National Cardiovascular Center in Osaka, revealed that urban Japanese children have higher cholesterol levels than their American counterparts.

These dietary changes have already led to sharp increases in coronary disease among Japanese adults. Studies by the Department of Pathology at Kyushu University in Fukuoka have shown that the number of coronary deaths has been increasing over the last 40 years, but is still lower than that found in autopsy cases in the United States. The full impact of these dietary changes on heart disease, according to Dr. Omae, will not be clear for another 20 years.

In a nationwide Japanese cooperative study of atherosclerosis in infants, children, and young adults, atherosclerotic changes were observed to begin developing during childhood. Cholesterol levels were strongly correlated with the extent of fatty streaks in 1,620 coronary arteries studied at the autopsies of young Japanese, ranging in ages from 1 month to 39 years. The authors of the 1988 report concluded that the prevention of coronary disease must begin during childhood.

Another report, by Drs. I. A. Kashani and P. R. Nader in 1986, reached the same conclusion. They wrote that, since eating habits in infancy establish the basis for lifetime eating habits, pediatricians can have a significant impact by encouraging a diet low in saturated fat. "There is, therefore, a clear-cut need for guidelines to the general pediatrician for a sensible, effective and specific, yet harmless and cost efficient, approach."

Japanese pediatricians may find that this will not be an easy task, since Western fast-food outlets are now proliferating rapidly in Japan. According to the *New York Times* article, McDonald's in 1993 reported that Japan was its largest overseas market; the chain had opened more than 1,000 restaurants in the country. Dozens of other high-fat fast-food restaurants are already following McDonald's lead.

Children in Hong Kong, Taiwan, and mainland China have all had increasing levels of fat in their diets since the 1950s. These three areas still have much less coronary disease than most Western countries—about one-fourth to one-eighth of that of the United States. However, according to a 1989 study by the Chinese University of Hong Kong, whereas coronary disease is now gradually decreasing in the United States and Europe, these three areas, with a population of 1.2 billion, are experiencing a sharp increase in the disease. The children who had first been exposed to the increased dietary fat are now old enough to be having their first heart attacks.

The U.N. Food and Agriculture Organization reported in 1994 that in the urban Chinese population there has been a fourfold increase in the rate of diabetes, obesity, and heart disease since 1957. Kentucky Fried Chicken, McDonald's, and Baskin Robbins have all reported record sales in their China outlets, reflecting the increasing fat taste in this country. McDonald's largest restaurant in the world, in Beijing, serves 10,000 customers a day. Lines are forming at 9:00 A.M., even though the restaurant doesn't serve breakfast. Considering the rural population, however, the average Chinese fat consumption remains 64 percent less than that of North Americans.

As parts of the world move from poverty to affluence, increases in children's dietary fat, cholesterol levels, and—ultimately—coronary disease are first seen in areas with the highest per-capita income. Mortality rates from coronary heart disease in Singapore, a city-state of more than 3 million with a per-capita income and population comparable to those of Los Angeles, have increased during the past two decades to levels found in America and England. This is almost certainly due to the sharp increase in dietary fat and cholesterol levels found in a 1989 survey by the Department of Community, Occupational, and Family Medicine at the National University Hospital in Singapore. The consumption of fat and blood-cholesterol levels among Singaporian children have reached levels similar to those in Western countries.

Answers from Asia

According to the China Health Study, the rural Chinese in the smaller villages have not had such an increase in dietary fat. This study, a joint research venture of the Chinese government, Cornell University, and Oxford University, was conducted over a six-year period beginning in 1983. One hundred individuals from each of 65 counties were studied. Measurements were made of 284 dietary and life-style characteristics in each of these 6,500 Chinese, who had typically lived in one village since chilldhood, traveling rarely, and eating food from local sources (in the United States, food is shipped an average of 1,200 miles before it's consumed). The raw material of the study, about 1,846,000 measurements, was published for the use of researchers studying the effects of diet and life-style on chronic diseases.

Far less coronary disease and cancer were found in the smaller Southern villages, where the fat intake was the lowest, 10–15 percent of calories. *The rate of heart disease—not death rate from heart disease, just the disease itself—in these rural villages of China was 26 per 100,000. The rate in the United States is 4,036 per 100,000 or 155 times higher.*

The mortality rate for breast cancer in rural China, for ages up to 64, was only one-sixth the British or American rate. This difference was even greater when comparing areas of China with the lowest fat consumption.

Codirector Dr. T. Colin Campbell found that the rural Chinese consumed one-third more calories per unit of body weight than did Americans, yet had 20 percent less body mass. He explains that obesity is far less common among Chinese than Americans, because of greater physical activity and the consumption of a low-fat, low-animal-protein diet. The Chinese blood-cholesterol levels ranged from a low of 100 in the smaller Southern villages to 190 in the North, where the fat consumption is greater. There was a difference of 10 times or more between the highest and lowest percentages of fat consumed in Chinese villages. The Chinese fiber intake, about 33 grams daily, was triple that of Americans.

European Diet "Americanized"

In European countries, children have adopted a higher-fat diet far more rapidly than those in Asia. This would be expected to lead to higher adult death rates from coronary heart disease.

The fat consumption of British children has usually matched that in the United States. In a study comparing a community in England where children's fat consumption was low with one where it was high, East Birmingham Hospital found sharp differences in adult coronary-heart-disease rates in the two communities.

The cholesterol levels of 15-to-16-year-old male students from schools of the community with low adult death rates from coronary heart disease were compared with those from schools in the community with high death rates. The schools with the highest cholesterol levels among its students were in the community with a rate of adult heart-attack deaths four times higher than that among adults in the community where children's cholesterol levels were lower. This is a recurrent finding throughout the world: children's eating habits lead to coronary disease which is not recognized until later in life.

Italian Diet "Americanized"

Other European countries, with a long history of consuming little fat, are now catching up to England and the United States. A report in the *International Journal of Cardiology* in 1990 described autopsy studies of 100 children, ages 1 to 20 in the Italian region of Veneto who had died from causes unrelated to the cardiovascular system. The children of northern Italy in general have increased their intake of dietary fat and have had higher cholesterol levels for the past several decades.

The researchers were startled when thickenings were found in the left anterior descending coronary artery, the main vessel supplying blood to the front of the left side of the heart, in *95.3 percent of the children ages 1 to 5.* Larger and thicker lesions, called *plaques,* were found in 15 of the children. These findings were unexpected, and the authors expressed alarm because of recent reports of sudden coronary deaths in young people from the same geographic area.

Children in the northern-Italian city of Milan were found to have a much higher fat intake, were heavier, and had higher blood-cholesterol levels than children in southern Italy. The Milanese children were similar in these respects to their counterparts in other Western countries, including the United States. This 1992 report also confirmed a higher intake of fat and higher cholesterol levels in children in cities where the typical diet is higher in fat.

As already mentioned, Finland, especially eastern Finland, has long been known to have the highest rate of coronary heart disease in the world. In recent years, however, Northern Ireland and Scotland have edged just above Finland for this "honor." It is interesting to note that, according to independent multinational studies done by Drs. Ernst Wynder and J. T. Knuiman, children in these nations have the highest cholesterol levels. However, a report published by Dr. J. Viikari, a researcher at the University of Turku (Finland), states that serum-cholesterol levels have decreased among Finns during the 1980s by about 1 percent per year. He added that this should lead to improvements in the nation's high rate of heart attacks in the future.

Increasing Dietary Fat in South America

I found similar evidence of children consuming increasing amounts of fat in areas within the "Fourth World" continents. In South America, where children have eaten a very low-fat diet for centuries, there are affluent groups in which elementary-school students are now eating as much high-fat food as their counterparts in the United States.

A study was done in Mérida, Venezuela, among children from private and public schools. These students' fat intake and cholesterol levels were compared with those of students of the Princeton School District in Cincinnati, Ohio. The report, in 1980, showed that Venezuelan children from private schools ingested more fat (almost twice as much) and had higher cholesterol levels than Venezuelan public-school children. The fat intake and cholesterol levels of the private students were comparable to those of public-school children in Cincinnati, Ohio. The Venezuelan private students also consumed more calories and more protein, and were heavier than the public-school students in Mérida.

The authors concluded that "Westernization" of affluent segments of Venezuelan society is associated with cholesterol levels that, if maintained into adulthood, would increase the risk of coronary heart disease to the same degree as in the United States.

Africans Are Eating More Fat

South Africa, a nation of another Fourth World continent where children have always eaten low-fat food, shows isolated signs that children and parents are now eating more fat. The Centre for Epidemiological Research in Southern Africa, writing in a 1990 report, identified 976 black subjects, including children, of the Cape Peninsula who consume a typical Western diet, with 37 percent of their calories from fat. Blood-cholesterol levels and incidence of coronary-artery disease were much higher in this group than among the people on the usual South African diet, containing far less fat.

These findings in South Africa are the first to show that the higher fat consumption—which had already led to a rise in cholesterol levels and an increase in heart disease of the Indian, colored, and white South Africans—may now be appearing in the black population.

As this vast body of proof mounts—that coronary heart disease and other chronic adult illnesses begin during childhood—it has not escaped the recent attention of health authorities at the local level and in both houses of Congress in our own country. For example, in Louisiana, where high dietary fat is a risk factor for the state's three leading causes of death—heart disease, cancer, and stroke—the Department of Public Health has issued a statement to all practicing physicians recommending efforts to influence children to sample and consume low-fat foods. The announcement, in the January 1993 issue of *Louisiana Morbidity Report*, stated that this would have a lifetime effect on their food preferences. And, as described on page 149, new federal legislation to reduce dietary fat in school lunches was passed in 1994.

A Major Source of Saturated Fat (For Calves Only)

It should be clear from these studies that high cholesterol levels of children in North and South America, Europe, Asia, and Africa have led to coronary-artery heart disease of the adults in these five continents. In several areas, this has been a relatively recent phenomenon, following an increase in the fat consumption of children. Since the chief saturated fat sources during childhood, after meat, are milk and dairy products, these must be reduced sharply or eliminated in order to prevent heart disease. This is a difficult decision for many parents.

In September 1992, representatives of the Physicians' Committee for Responsible Medicine (PCRM) held a press conference in Boston, in which the group's president, Dr. Neal Barnard, of George Washington University, and Dr. Frank Oski, chief of pediatrics at Johns Hopkins University—representing the committee's approximately 3,000 physician-members—spoke out against all consumption of cow's milk during infancy and childhood. They cited the growing evidence that it causes lifelong allergies, coronary heart disease, cancer, and even insulin-dependent diabetes.

Dr. Oski said, "There is no redeeming feature to cow's milk that should make people drink it." Interviewed by *The Wall Street Journal*, he added, "It was designed for calves, not humans."

Alongside them stood Dr. Benjamin Spock, who feels that cow's milk is nutritionally unacceptabale during infancy (after the child has been weaned from breast milk). Dr. Spock, however, did *not* join the committee in saying that cow's milk is unsafe for *older* children.

Dr. Ronald E. Kleinman, chairman of the American Academy of Pediatrics' Committee on Nutrition, called this "nutritional terrorism" in an interview with *The New York Times*. "The major problem with their position is that they are unnecessarily frightening parents who worry that they will do harm if they continue to allow their children to have dairy products." He went on to say that pediatricians should trust the advice they have been giving for the last 100 years.

During the last 100 years, however, coronary-artery disease has become the nation's number-one killer; before the turn of the century, it wasn't among the top 10 causes of death.

I strongly agree with the PCRM position. It's a necessary first step in reducing total fat, and especially saturated fat, in the diets of children. During my years of practice, I have observed the damaging effects of cow's milk in 7 out of 10 of my patients. It causes anemia, and allergic disorders such as asthma, eczema, and sinusitis, and it is the single largest source of saturated fat in children's diets.

Also present at the PCRM news conference was Suzanne Havala, a registered dietitian from North Carolina and primary author of "Position of the American Dietetic Association: Vegetarian Diets." She stated that, after weaning, there is no need for milk of any sort. "Generally, if a vegetarian child is getting enough calories and reasonable variety in his diet, then he should be able to get enough calcium (and riboflavin) from plant foods without drinking milk or taking supplements." She went on to say that the officially recommended daily need for calcium is set much higher than a human's true requirement to compensate for the American high-protein diet.

A Low-Fat Mandate for Children

These numerous studies discussed above should give the NIH, the AHA, and the AAP a clear mandate to recommend *further meaningful reductions* in children's dietary fat. Their guidelines, however, appear to be fixed for the foreseeable future. Meanwhile, heart disease is still appearing during early childhood and progressing, gradually and silently, into adulthood, where it is finally, and often fatally, taken seriously.

Chapter 19

Summit in the Desert

The public do not know enough to be experts,
yet know enough to decide between them.
—*Samuel Butler (1835–1901)*

*I*n October 1991, with no likely official change of guidelines on the horizon, a surgeon at the Cleveland Clinic convinced an elite panel of nutritional scientists to meet with concerned practicing physicians from across the nation at a remote Arizona resort. At this "summit meeting," their ideas and research findings were exchanged and a general consensus was reached that children and adults should consume less dietary fat than was recommended by the NIH and the AHA. I was invited to the gathering as a physician-journalist to report the proceedings to a group of 30 Louisiana newspapers.

Dr. Caldwell B. Esselstyn, Jr., a thyroid surgeon at the Cleveland Clinic, where coronary bypass surgery was pioneered more than 30 years ago, questioned this traditional treatment approach to coronary-artery disease. The disease, he said to his colleagues during the planning stages of the conference, must be prevented, rather than treated by surgery and high-tech coronary care—an unusual approach by a surgeon. He pointed to the mounting evidence that heart disease actually starts in childhood and is the direct result of excessive saturated fat in the diet.

The Desert Meeting

It was an ambitious project, but under the sponsorship of the Caldwell B. Esselstyn Foundation—established in 1976 in memory of Dr. Esselstyn's father, Caldwell Blakemen Esselstyn, M.D., an early pioneer in HMOs—the 1st National Conference on the Elimination of Coronary Artery Disease was held at Loews Ventana Canyon Resort, outside Tucson, Arizona.

In order to avoid any possibility of bias in the conclusions reached by the scientists, the usual special-interest sponsorships were declined: no drug-company funding or federal grants were accepted. The conference was, in Dr. Esselstyn's words, "unadulterated"; the entire cost was covered by the foundation and fees were paid by 50 attending physicians, to whom educational credits for attending the meeting were granted by the Cleveland Clinic Foundation.

The panel members were:

Gerald S. Berenson, M.D., Professor, Department of Medicine; Chief, Section of Cardiology, Louisiana State University Medical Center; Director, Bogalusa Heart Study.

T. Colin Campbell, Ph.D., Jacob Gould Schurman Professor of Nutritional Biochemistry, Division of Nutritional Sciences; Project Director, China Project on Nutrition, Environment and Health, Cornell University.

William P. Castelli, M.D., Director, Framingham Heart Study, National Heart, Lung and Blood Institute, National Institutes of Health.

Harold T. Dodge, M.D., Professor of Medicine, Department of Medicine, University of Washington.

James F. Fries, M.D., Associate Professor of Medicine, Division of Immunology and Rheumatology, Stanford University School of Medicine.

Alexander Leaf, M.D., Ridley Watts Professor, Preventive Medicine, Harvard Medical School.

Dean Ornish, M.D., President and Director, Preventive Medicine Research Institute; Assistant Clinical Professor of Medicine, School of Medicine, University of California.

Thomas A. Ports, M.D., Professor of Medicine; Director, Cardiac Catheterization Laboratories, Cardiovascular Research Institute, University of California.

Miguel E. Sanmarco, M.D., Associate Professor of Clinical Medicine, University of Southern California.

Renu Virmani, M.D., Chairperson, Department of Cardiovascular Pathology, Armed Forces Institute of Pathology; Clinical Professor, Department of Pathology, Georgetown University.

Ernst L. Wynder, M.D., President and Medical Director, American Health Foundation; Clinical Professor of Community and Preventive Medicine, New York Medical College.

Ronald Hart, M.D., Director of the National Center of Toxological Research, National Institutes of Health.

Basil M. Rifkind, M.D., Chief, Lipid Metabolism–Atherogenesis Branch, Division of Heart and Vascular Diseases, National Heart, Lung and Blood Institute, National Institutes of Health.

It was a unique gathering, with attendees seeming to practice the same life-style they recommended for their patients. I've attended hundreds of medical conferences and usually find that physicians eat typical high-fat American food. Not here. According to the hotel's restaurants, there were more requests for vegetarian meals than at any other time in its history. The panel and attending doctors were also atypical in other respects: most had devoted a major part of their professional careers to the practice of preventive, rather that curative, medicine.

A Strong Consensus Prevailed

Incredibly, 11 of the 13 scientists on the panel, even though they took differing approaches—through statistics, population studies, clinical trials, and animal studies—all reached the same conclusion: *not only is the typical American diet for children and adults much too high in fat, animal protein, and calories, but the guideline of the NIH and the AHA, recommending up to 30 percent of calories from fat, is not low enough.* Also, several of their studies showed actual progression of existing coronary-artery disease among people on the officially recommended diet.

The ideal diet, nearly everyone agreed, is plant-based, with little or no animal products, deriving only 10–15 percent of its calories from fat. And the ideal time to start such a diet is during childhood, before a taste for fat is fully developed.

The China Health Study

Dr. T. Colin Campbell, nutritional biochemist from Cornell, presented results from his China Health Study, showing far less coronary heart disease and cancer among Chinese who had consumed a diet of vegetables and grains, with little or no meat or dairy products. This study, described in the last chapter, was conducted on adults but had strong implications for children's eating patterns, *since 95 percent of the study subjects had lived in the same village and eaten the same locally grown food since birth.*

Reversing Coronary Disease

Most of us at the desert conference knew that we all had varying degrees of *invisible* coronary disease already. After all, the Chinese children may be eating the ideal diet to prevent coronary disease, but we had all eaten a typical American diet during our childhood. "But what about us Americans [60–80 million adults] who already have this disease?" someone asked. "Since we didn't prevent it during our youth, what do we do now?"

Fortunately, the situation isn't hopeless. Dr. Dean Ornish told us about his study—the subject of his two books, *Dr. Dean Ornish's Program for Reversing Heart Disease* and *Eat More, Weigh Less*—showing that a vegetarian diet, without animal products (except egg whites and nonfat dairy products), reducing cholesterol levels to below 150, can actually reverse coronary-artery disease without bypass surgery. Furthermore, *the control subjects in his study, who followed the American Heart Association guidelines (up to 30 percent of calories from fat, and 10 percent from saturated fat), had progression of their coronary disease*. Ornish recommended that fat be reduced to 10 percent of calories in order to reverse coronary heart disease.

I had originally met Dr. Ornish at the 1988 First National Cholesterol Conference, in Washington, D.C. His ideas were simply unacceptable at the time to the NIH, the organization that was sponsoring the meeting. Now, three years later, he had proved his case in clinical trials. He showed us slides of coronary-artery obstructions before and after a strict vegetarian diet, with undeniable regression. There was no more skepticism from NIH officials.

Even more meaningful acceptance was still to come. On July 28, 1993, *The New York Times* reported that Mutual of Omaha would now cover expenses involved in the Ornish Plan; insurance companies had not covered preventive diet plans prior to this. The cost of the Ornish Plan for individuals with coronary heart disease in 1993 dollars was $3,500 a year, about one-tenth the cost of conventional coronary care. As a result, medical facilities throughout the country began setting up Ornish-type clinics, where people were treated with a very low-fat diet, moderate exercise, and stress-control measures such as relaxation and meditation.

The people in Dr. Ornish's studies were adults who already had heart disease. A similar diet program, in his opinion, is appropriate for children over the age of 2 for primary prevention of this disease.

Others on the panel, including Dr. Berenson, agreed that children should be on the same low-fat diet as adults.

Dr. Ernst Wynder challenged the other 12 panelists to reach a consensus during the following two days, something on which the public could rely. Dr. Wynder was passionate in his plea to us that we stand and be counted among those who support greater reductions in dietary fat than those recommended by the NIH and the AHA. It was impossible not to reminisce about his equally passionate (and lonely) stand against tobacco 42 years ago.

Coronary Disease Isn't Found Everywhere

Dr. William Castelli, director of the Framingham Study, pointed out, as discussed in Chapter 1, that our leading killer is unknown among 75 percent of the people on this planet, who have not been exposed to our high-fat, high-protein food. For example, the rural Chinese, even though 80 percent of the men smoke, have an average cholesterol level of about 100–120 and suffer practically no coronary disease. Most members of the panel thought that this could be achieved in a nation of affluence like the United States only by reducing the dietary fat to 10–15 percent of calories from early childhood on, thereby keeping the cholesterol level below 150.

As mentioned in Chapter 1, Dr. Castelli said, *"We've never had a heart attack in Framingham in anyone with a cholesterol level under 150.* Dr. Alexander Leaf added that, with our present knowledge, 70–80 percent of coronary heart disease could be prevented, reducing heart attacks from 1.5 million to 300,000 and the resulting deaths from 500,000 to 100,000 per year.

Dairy Products Unpopular

The high saturated-fat content of dairy products was repeatedly referred to by the panelists during their presentations. The general agreement was that nonfat milk and other dairy products were acceptable, but that 2-percent milk—designated low-fat by the dairy industry, with federal approval—contains too much fat (35 percent of its calories). A clinical dietitian reminded the panel and attending doctors that (as discussed in Chapter 7) no other animals drink milk after weaning, yet they all maintain strong bones and do not develop osteoporosis.

Elderly Mice

Two panel members had applied dietary changes to laboratory animals. Since human studies all suggest that a longer, healthier life may result from preventing coronary heart disease and many cancers, one would expect that studies of animals, whose life spans are shorter, might answer some of our questions about diet and longevity. Dr. Ronald Hart, director of the National Center for Toxicological Research, and Cornell's Dr. Campbell described their current independent studies on mice. Dr. Hart's mice had fewer tumors and lived 50 percent longer on a diet of reduced total calories. The mice finally just died suddenly, disease-free.

Dr. Campbell's mice showed the same reduction of tumors and increased life span when fed a diet with greatly reduced animal protein or with reduced fat, but with no restriction of carbohydrate calories.

Similar studies had been reported in the past. Dr. Roy Walford, a pathologist and researcher on aging at UCLA, substantially extended the life span of mice with a low-calorie, low-protein, low-fat diet in 1980. And in 1952, at Cornell University, Dr. Cleve McCay was able to *double* the life span of rats by restricting calories and fat. Therefore, for more than 40 years, animal studies seem to have confirmed the conclusions from concurrent human clinical trials: that reduced calories from fat prevent some of the most serious chronic degenerative diseases.

By the end of the meeting, it was clear that almost all of the panelists and attending physicians believed that the current national guidelines weren't low enough. Dr. Campbell summarized the group's opinion:

If we are reasonably sure of what our data from these studies are telling us, then why must we be reticent about recommending a diet which we know is safe and healthy? We, as scientists, can no longer take the attitude that the public cannot benefit from information they are not ready for.

We must have the integrity to tell them the truth and let them decide what to do with it. We cannot force them to follow the guidelines we recommend, but we can give them these guidelines and then let them decide. I personally have great faith in the public.

We must tell them that a diet of roots, stems, seeds, flowers, fruit, and leaves is the healthiest diet and the only diet we can promote, endorse, and recommend.

A Consensus from the Conference

A resolution was prepared to cover the opinions and recommendations which I have paraphrased here. The exact resolution is awaiting publication by Dr. Esselstyn as part of another clinical study in progress.

The strong opinion of the panel was that the current national guidelines for fat and saturated-fat consumption would not prevent coronary-artery disease. They pointed out—as we have already discussed in Chapter 4—that people who already have coronary disease experience a *progression* of it while following these guidelines.

The panel felt that an ideal diet for preventing, arresting, and reversing coronary disease would be one deriving 10–15 percent of calories from fat, consisting of vegetables, fruits, grains, and legumes. This kind of diet, they said, has also been shown to reduce the risk of cancer of the breast, colon, prostate, and ovary. It is, in their opinion, safe, and adequate in vitamins and minerals.

It was the panel's opinion that a diet such as this was safe for children over the age of 2, and should be introduced early for the development of proper eating habits and optimal nutrition. They suggested that schools have the unique opportunity to promote such a low-fat diet.

The affluent Western high-fat diet, said the panel, has spawned an epidemic of heart disease and cancer. Therefore, they feel that the medical profession should recommend to the public a diet that protects them from these diseases.

Finally, the panel agreed that the American people have a right to know the facts about their dietary risk; they must be informed and will decide for themselves.

The consensus resolution covering all of these topics was endorsed and signed by 10 of the 13 panel members present at the conference.

Chapter 20

How You're Misinformed

> I should have no objection to a repetition of the
> same life from its beginning, only asking the
> advantage authors have in a second edition to
> correct some faults of the first.
> —*Benjamin Franklin*
> *(1706–90)*

> Truth is the most valuable thing we have, let us
> encourage it.
> —*Mark Twain*
> *(1835–1910)*

> Telling the truth to people who misunderstand
> you is generally promoting falsehood.
> —*Anthony Hawkins (1863–1933)*
> *British author*

*S*cientific facts have, in recent years, been reported to the public
—including practicing physicians, dietitians, and legislators—in a
way that misrepresents them. Often this has involved mistakes in
interpreting scientific reports; on other occasions, the truth was
reported, but was tainted to prove another point. As said best by
eighteenth-century physicist G. C. Lichtenberg, "The most dangerous of all falsehoods is a slightly distorted truth."

One of the latest ideas making the rounds, even among medically informed people, is the myth that, if all coronary heart disease were prevented, a person's life span would increase only by about 3 years. When the media reported this, based on an article in the American Heart Association journal *Circulation* in April 1991, its effect was enormously discouraging for thousands of people who were making a sincere effort to improve their diets. Physicians began telling their patients, "Relax and enjoy yourself."

Gain Only 8 Months?

The *Circulation* article, with the impressive title "Expected Gains in Life Expectancy from Various Coronary Heart Disease Risk Factor Modifications," used computer projections for the U.S. population to show that, among 35-year-old men, reducing their cholesterol levels to 200 would extend their lives by only 8 months. For women, the extension was about 9 months. Eliminating coronary heart disease entirely, they wrote, would extend the average life expectancy of a 35-year-old man by 3.1 years and 3.3 years for women. Their conclusion: "gains in life expectancy from risk factor modification are modest."

This misleading and damaging report was taking into account *all* deaths from *all* causes in the *entire* U.S. population, including those that were not preventable and those individuals who were not likely to develop heart disease. However, they failed to point out to the reader that, *of those individuals who would have died prematurely of coronary heart disease, life would have been extended much longer—12.4 years, according to the National Center for Health Statistics*. Also, the reduction of serum cholesterol to 200 is a very modest improvement, not enough to stop completely plaque formation within coronary arteries. As discussed, *stopping plaque formation requires a drop in cholesterol levels to 150 or below.*

Following the extensive media reports of this article, many of my colleagues phased out their already meager efforts to reduce their patients' dietary fat. At a hospital staff meeting in my community, the unofficial consensus among the physicians was, "Now maybe everyone will quit bugging us about their cholesterol!" I had heard some of them complain that parents were overly concerned about reducing their children's dietary fat. Parents have always taken this far more seriously than have their family doctors. For example, a 1989 survey by the AHA revealed that *more patients than physicians were of the opinion that elevated cholesterol levels caused coronary disease.* Even today, I overheard a physician in my community hospital's emergency room say that he had patients who believed in this "cholesterol thing."

Cardiologists Are Back on Bacon Burgers

Reports such as the one in *Circulation,* widely quoted in the media, may also have an impact upon the eating habits of practicing physicians, who should be setting an example for their patients. It should be obvious that credibility cannot be maintained by such primary-care doctors unless they can follow the life-style pattern they recommend for their patients.

For example, many of the 30,000 doctors, nurses, and researchers at the 1993 annual meeting of the American Heart Association, according to an Associated Press report, "talk healthy diets out of one side of their mouth and put burgers and fries in the other." They were seen by the dozens eating Big Bacon Classic Burgers and Biggie Fries at a Wendy's near the convention site. When asked if this set a bad example, a cardiologist from Charlotte, North Carolina, said that he removed his name tag while eating fatty food at the conference.

These were apparently not just isolated reports. "Fast food is just as popular among those at the heart association meeting as it is with people at other conventions," said Jane Jaeger, director of sales and marketing for the convention-hall caterer.

Since physicians, even cardiologists, are not taking their own diets seriously, I'm convinced that first the consumer—you and your children—must be educated, and the health professional will follow. Meanwhile, the debate continues about the advantages of a low-fat diet.

Dr. Walter Bortz, a preventive cardiologist at Stanford University, estimated in his book *We Live Too Short and Die Too Long* that, based on his experiences, if all arteriosclerosis were eliminated, a person 65 years old could accrue from 10 to 16 years of additional life.

Misrepresentations of other medical-risk modifications have occurred. For example, a report on the years of life gained by quitting smoking was published by the Harvard Medical School in the *American Journal of Medicine* in July 1992. The average 35-year-old man, they wrote, would live only 2.3 years longer if he quit smoking, and total smoking cessation in this country would increase the American life span by approximately a year. When, however, the life extension of an *individual* smoker is considered, those who would have died of coronary heart disease or lung cancer because of smoking live many years longer. Estimates among scientists range up to 18 years. Reporting risk modifications based on total populations is meaningless and can be of interest only to statisticians. The media have simply misinterpreted these studies.

Another example of how statistics can be misunderstood by the public is seen in cancer reports. The National Center for Health Statistics reported that, if all breast cancer were eliminated, the average American woman would live only 7 months longer. Again, this took into consideration the entire female population, including millions of women who never get breast cancer. The extension of life of the individual women who would have died of breast cancer would be 17 years.

A far more accurate indication of how life-style habits may affect health and longevity is seen in a 20-year study reported in 1993 in the journal *Preventive Medicine*. Beginning in 1972, several life-style habits were examined. Men who showed an increase of 11 years of additional life among 7,000 residents of Alameda County, California, were nonsmokers, moderate exercisers, of normal weight, had moderate alcohol intake, ate regular meals, and slept 7 or 8 hours a night. Twenty years later, the same researcher, Dr. Lester Breslow, a California public-health specialist, reported again on his 7,000 subjects. Those with the above life-style habits, who had escaped death were also found through follow-up surveys to be more likely to live out their lives without chronic illness and disability.

It is reasonable to assume that there is even greater potential for better health and life extension than that achieved by these moderate health rules if, during childhood, cholesterol and obesity are controlled by proper reductions in dietary fat.

However, despite the growing body of evidence, arguments by well-meaning writers still appear in major medical journals for keeping children on their typical high-fat American diets. As already discussed, the reasons are primarily based on the unfounded fears of possible growth retardation and malnutrition.

The following conclusion was printed (in June 1992) in the *Journal of the American College of Nutrition:* "Strict adherence to low-fat, low-cholesterol diets in childhood may result in nutritional growth failure, while long-term benefits in reducing coronary heart disease may not be accomplished for the majority of the population who may not need marked dietary changes. Moderation is the theme for adequate nutrition in childhood."

Once again, moderation means different eating patterns for different cultures. In rural Japan and China, as I have already discussed, a moderate diet is usually accompanied by cholesterol levels below 150, with almost no future risk of heart disease. In America, a moderate diet leads to high cholesterol levels in at least one-third of all children, which leads to heart disease as adults.

> The rural Japanese's or Chinese's moderate diet is healthful. American moderation has proved deadly.

Truthful, but Misleading

Another report that was misinterpreted by the media and the public was published by the Louisiana State University Medical Center in 1993. When 871 10-year-old grade-schoolers were studied, those who consumed less than 30 percent of their calories from fat had lower intakes of B12, thiamin, and niacin. However, these weren't children whose parents and schools had *intentionally* reduced their fat intake; most were poor, malnourished children with *no* nutritional guidance. Parents and professionals who read about the LSU studies in the popular press were not made aware of this. Studies have failed to find significant clinical signs of B-vitamin deficiencies among rural Chinese, who consume *less* than 10 percent of calories from fat.

Media reports of scientific studies are often misleading because the studies are misunderstood. In the spring of 1993, I read four different newspaper accounts of a new study done at the University of Minnesota's Heart Disease Prevention Clinic. The findings, published in the *New England Journal of Medicine,* had shown a very slight (5-percent) reduction in cholesterol among people placed on the American Heart Association's Step II diet—a reduction of *saturated* fat to 7 percent of calories. *The New York Times, The Wall Street Journal,* and the *Denver Post* all implied that the low-fat diet wasn't effective until the drug Mevacor was given, at which point the cholesterol fell 27 percent. Only the *Rocky Mountain News* correctly pointed out that the study was financed by Merck & Co., the makers of Mevacor, and that the diets were poorly controlled. None of the papers pointed out that the AHA Step II diet allows 30 percent of calories from fat and that many researchers feel that this amount of fat reduction isn't enough to produce meaningful reductions in cholesterol levels.

The *Rocky Mountain News* and the *Minneapolis Star-Tribune* responsibly quoted Dr. P. J. Palumbo, the Mayo Clinic's leading expert on cholesterol, as saying that the study could be misleading and he feared it would drive people back to higher-fat diets. He pointed out that several surveys had shown that Americans were ignoring dietary advice and had returned to high-fat diets. The result, he said, would be a reversal in the hard-earned downward trend in heart disease in this country.

His concern is well founded. A nationwide poll reported in the May 1993 issue of the *Tufts University Diet & Nutrition Letter* revealed that 51 percent of Americans said they try hard to avoid fat, down from 58 percent in 1989.

Other polls would seem to confirm this. According to *Prevention* magazine's eleventh annual study of America's preventive health behaviors: in 1994, 52 percent of adults said they were working to cut fat in their diets, down from 58 percent in 1993 and 57 percent in 1992.

Yet another pollster agrees that the decades-long trend toward healthier life-styles has taken a turn for the worse. According to a December 1994 Louis Harris poll, more Americans were eating less carefully than in 1983. As a result, 69 percent were overweight, up from 66 percent in 1992 and 58 percent in 1983.

Is a Low Cholesterol Level Risky?

Perhaps the most striking example of misinformation to reach the general public is a report in the journal *Circulation* by the National Heart, Lung, and Blood Institute (a division of the NIH) in the summer of 1992. After examining the findings of 19 international trials involving 300,000 men and women, they reported that people with very low cholesterol levels (under 160) had four times the risk of dying of suicide, alcoholism, chronic obstructive lung disease, cerebral hemorrhage, or cancer of the lung, liver, or pancreas.

Another 1992 report, in the *Archives of Internal Medicine,* described the findings of a 12-year study of more than 350,000 healthy men. The 6 percent of these men who had very low cholesterol levels were twice as likely to die of cerebral hemorrhage, three times as likely to die of liver cancer, five times as likely to die from alcoholism, and twice as likely to commit suicide. Both reports were widely reported in newspapers across the nation, with predictable results: abandonment of already fragile life-style improvements.

The flaw in these two studies is that very low cholesterol levels in individuals on the average *moderate* American diet, which is high in saturated fat, are often a sign of unknown chronic disease, like cancer or chronic lung disease, which in turn may likely be associated with alcoholism or suicide. The very low cholesterol levels among Japanese and Chinese children and adults who are on low-fat diets are not associated with more deaths from cancer, lung disease, alcoholism, or suicide. Their rates for these disorders are *much less* than those in Western countries.

If these studies were examined in terms of individuals *on low-fat diets* with low cholesterol levels and a young-adult age group with low cholesterol levels, they would yield findings of very low death rates, not only from heart disease, but also from cancer, alcholism, and suicide.

For more reassurance about the safety of reducing cholesterol levels, we must turn to impeccable sources, such as the large clinical trials spanning several decades. For example, in 45 years of follow-up of 4,374 people in the Framingham Study, and in 361,662 individuals in the MRFIT trials (the large diet-intervention study reported during the mid-1980s), the association between low cholesterol levels and cancer was thought to be due to the cholesterol-lowering effects of unrecognized cancer or other chronic diseases.

Even the National Heart, Lung, and Blood Institute members who conducted the study reported in *Circulation* believed that low cholesterol itself was not the cause of the cancer, alcholism, and suicide deaths. They thought the low cholesterol levels were the *result* of underlying undiagnosed diseases. But this is not the way the mass media reported the findings. Once again, the public was misled.

Further evidence of this came in 1993 with the 19-year follow-up reports of the Chicago Heart Association studies. These showed that there was no relationship between low cholesterol levels and death from violent causes such as suicide. The researchers concluded that a low cholesterol level was a "marker" of unrecognized cancer, cirrhosis, and hemorrhagic stroke and not a cause of these diseases. Again, the articles in *Circulation* and the *Archives of Internal Medicine* were the only ones reported by the media to the public. The Chicago Heart Association studies, reported in the journal *Cardiology* remained largely unknown outside scientific circles.

This effect of chronic, unrecognized disease is further understood when we look at the cholesterol levels of young, healthy individuals. As discussed on page 156, the 1993 Johns Hopkins study of 20-year-olds, followed for 42 years, showed *no* increased risk of death from cancer, accidents, strokes, or suicide in those with very low cholesterol. Once again this suggests that the 1992 reports described above were flawed: they included the elderly and were measuring depressed cholesterol levels from silent, pre-existing diseases.

The facts reported in the two scientific reports in *Circulation* and the *Archives of Internal Medicine* were accurate but misunderstood by the media and the public. However, within months, several respected experts in the fields of nutrition and preventive medicine called for a moratorium on universal screening for cholesterol and dietary restriction of fat in people with no symptoms of heart disease. This was a frightening thought, considering that, in one-third of people with coronary-artery disease, the first symptom, a heart attack, leads to death!

Dr. Stephen Hulley, of the University of California at San Francisco, suggested in 1992 that cholesterol levels no longer be checked in women. This was especially disturbing since women die of coronary-artery disease in numbers equal to men, and women are more likely to die from their first heart attack, because they are not diagnosed early. In March 1993, Dr. Hulley's article in the *Journal of the American Medical Association* stated that we should abandon all cholesterol testing in young adults except those who already have coronary disease, several risk factors, or a parent or sibling with a herditary cholesterol problem.

As for children, Dr. Hulley and his colleague, pediatrician Dr. Thomas Newman, said in an interview with the *Denver Post*: "Cholesterol measurement and therapy should be directed at the high-risk population, not at kids." They went on to say, "There are adverse effects to telling children and their parents that they are at high risk of dying, especially when that risk is 50 years away." They added that calling children's attention to their cholesterol level may cause emotional disorders. I would compare this to ignoring the dangerous effects of smoking and obesity because many years lapse before the health problems they cause appear.

Suzanne Bennett Johnson, a clinical psychologist at the University of Florida at Gainesville, disagrees: "Within three months, people adapt and go on with their lives. The anxiety level returns to normal." After her father and husband had a heart attack, her 10-year-old daughter's cholesterol level was tested and found to be high.

The psychologist said that whatever anxiety the cholesterol testing caused in her daughter was a good motivational force to get her to change her diet.

So to stop cholesterol testing these "low-risk" groups would be unwise. Young men and premenopausal women, like children, have a lower *short-term* risk for heart disease than do older persons—a heart attack may be many years in the future—but if this disease is to be prevented, the long-term risk is where our attention should be. A lower-fat diet and cholesterol testing are therefore necessary for children, young adults, and premenopausal women, who usually already have early stages of coronary-artery disease. These measures will prevent its further progress and lead to healthier life-style behaviors.

Articles in respected medical journals in other countries are also vulnerable to misinterpretation and quickly spread beyond their national boundaries. The Department of Epidemiology and Population Sciences of the London School of Hygiene and Tropical Medicine placed such a report in the British journal *Lancet* in 1990. They concluded that a lower level of cholesterol, which is associated with a longer life, is expected to reduce the lifetime risk of fatal heart disease, but people would then die of other diseases. This was obvious, since people eventually die of something, but was interpreted by the media to mean that controlling cholesterol and coronary disease does not prolong life or enhance health.

Starting Early May Save Money

Beginning during the early 1990s, reports began appearing in scientific journals questioning the cost-effectiveness of reducing cholesterol by diet or drugs or both. When these appeared in the public media, many readers found it difficult to understand. A Norwegian study, reported in May 1991 by the Institute of Community Medicine of the University of Troms, projected that the cost of lowering cholesterol based on individual dietary changes was £12,400 (about $18,500 at the time of the study) per person per life-year gained. This included the educational cost for promoting healthier eating habits among the population. The estimate is probably correct when applied to the population at large, including all the individuals who would never have died of coronary disease.

It has since become popular to calculate educational, drug, and promotional cost in this manner. Judith Walsh, M.D., of the Veterans Affairs Medical Center in San Francisco, wrote in 1993 that cholesterol testing and control with drugs and diet in young men cost $1 million per year of life saved. Again, though these calculations— which include our total population of young men, two-thirds of whom would not have died of coronary disease, and incurred the high cost of cholesterol-lowering drugs—are probably accurate, such reporting may be discouraging when conveyed in this context to the public. Yet, when Harvard's Center for Risk Analysis calculated the cost per year of life saved by cholesterol-testing 10-year-old boys in 1994, they came up with the bargain price of $6,500.

It *is* expensive to change the eating habits of adults by national educational programs. The use of cholesterol-reducing drugs in some high-risk adults adds even more to the expense. Children, however, with individual guidance from knowledgeable parents, can establish the proper diet at essentially no cost. Furthermore, the cost of low-fat, near-vegetarian food is much less than that of a typical Western diet. A research nutritionist at George Washington University calculated that, for a family of 4, a menu based on vegetables, fruit, grains, and legumes would cost only $40 per week, in 1992 dollars. Dr. Neal Barnard points out that this saves about $2,100 per year, enough to buy a new small car every 6 or 7 years.

Other studies have calculated similar savings. Researchers at the Mary Imogene Bassett Research Institute in Cooperstown, New York, for instance, found that people who decreased their intake of saturated fat and cholesterol saved an average of $1.00 per day. For a family of 4, this amounts to approximately $1,500 per year.

Misinterpretation Trumpeted to the Public

Bad dietary habits are sometimes inadvertently suggested to the public by highly credible people. Dr. William Nolen, author of the best-seller *The Making of a Surgeon,* wrote in his last book, *Crisis Time!* (1984), that one should not worry about changing dietary habits in order to live a few months longer. Regarding diet and weight control, "If you love rich desserts, even if it raises the likelihood of your dying a year earlier than you would otherwise by 1 percent, it's worth it to you."

Dr. Nolen's father had died of coronary disease at 58, his brother at 61. He would probably live longer than this, he told his readers, because modern drugs such as lovastatin, beta-blockers, and surgical procedures were now able to take care of heart disease. Describing a conference where he and low-fat-diet advocate Nathan Pritikin sat at the same dinner table, he wrote, "I'd already had my first coronary bypass at the time, and I was eating and enjoying meat, potatoes, and vegetables with ice cream for dessert. All Pritikin ate was a bunch of grapes. If I have to eat grapes for lunch to live possibly an extra six months, I'll pass."

"Why, Bill," I asked him at a conference in 1985, when he was 56 years old, "don't you take better care of yourself?" I pointed out that these marginal benefits in added life were based on total population studies, but for him, already at high risk for dying from coronary disease, a proper low-fat diet might extend his life by 20 years. He had just had his second coronary bypass operation at the time.

He merely said that if he really believed this he would do it, but he couldn't make the sacrifice, given so many reports showing such meager benefits. His inability to make changes, despite his high risk of heart disease, illustrates again why I feel that low-fat eating habits should be developed during childhood. Had Bill done this, he wouldn't have been facing such a hopeless prospect.

Millions of readers have been influenced by Dr. Nolen's six books and monthly column in *McCall's* magazine. Many are parents, who must make important decisions about their diets and those of their children. Many are physicians who must advise their patients about diet and life-style. For every reader of scientific studies by researchers such as Drs. Ornish, Campbell, and Castelli, there are hundreds who read books like Dr. Nolen's for the general public. Bill died in 1986 of a massive heart attack, at age 57.

A Decade of Education Vanishes

These flawed studies and misleading media reports have had a predictable effect on the diets of Americans, especially children and teenagers. Dr. Susan Calvert Finn, president of the American Dietetic Association, commented on the new signs of a nutritional backlash noted by her association. She said that a 1993 survey showed that only 39 percent of people are making an all-out effort to eat properly—down from 44 percent in 1991. One of the chief reasons given was confusion.

More evidence of a drift back toward high-fat foods is found in a 1993 report from Cornell University. Among surveyed women, poultry is eaten fried or breaded 71 percent of the time, and pork is eaten untrimmed and fried or breaded 68 percent of the time. These same women were found to consume inadequate quantities of fruits, vegetables, and fiber-rich grains. The backlash among children and teenagers, already discussed in Myth Five, who are returning to the higher-fat fast-food selections, is even more disturbing.

You are now empowered to reverse this perilous trend. The new wisdom you have acquired should "trickle up" to your physicians and educators. This is the way the medical profession finally learned about the urgent need to control smoking and hypertension. I believe that you, as a parent, once you've considered the evidence I've presented in this book, will instinctively make the right decisions.

> How can I teach, how can I save,
> This child whose features are my own,
> Whose feet run down the ways where
> I have walked.
> —*Michael Roberts (1902–48)*
> *British author*

Part Four

Helpful Hints, Menus, and Children-Tested Recipes

Chapter 21

A Mom's Guide to
Happy, Low-Fat Kids

BY VICTORIA MORAN

*W*hen I was pregnant with my daughter, I prayed that she would not have an insatiable sweet tooth, as I did as a child. My love of candy, cookies, pastries, and ice cream had made me an overweight youngster, with all the teasing and pain that can bring. Interestingly, my little girl *didn't* go for sweets. On the healthful diet I tried hard to provide, she progressed from mother's milk to solids with an eagerness to try new foods, but even as a toddler she preferred celery sticks to cookies, baked-potato fingers to candy. For her third birthday, she asked if we could put the candles in fruit instead of on a cake!

Then came the fateful day: We were eating at a restaurant and I suggested she try French fries. I figured that, with the whole-food, vegetarian diet we ate at home, she should be familiar with all-American fast foods to be prepared for the times she'd go out with her friends. (She was *3*, mind you. Only a first-time parent is concerned about peer pressure with a 3-year-old!) To say that the fries were a hit was to put it mildly. Rachael lost all interest in other foods until she could go out again and have more "Fwench fwies."

At that time, the dangers of dietary fat were less commonly known than they are today, so my concern with her fry fetish was not so much due to their fat content but because her craving for them was displacing other, more nutritious foods from her diet. The problem did encourage me to study the issue in more depth—a natural thing to do, since I'm a health writer by profession. That was when I first learned of the problems inherent in excess fat, even vegetable oils—problems that were as important for my preschooler to avoid as for her cholesterol-conscious grandparents.

The real epiphany of my research was that my own childhood bane, the sweet tooth, was less a matter of craving sugar than of craving fat. Pastries and ice cream are high-fat foods, just like fatty meats and cheeses, fried foods, nuts, whole milk, and butter. I hadn't gotten fat from eating hard candies and sugar cubes; I'd gotten fat from eating fat. My preference had been for the sweetened fat of desserts. My daughter had gravitated to the salted fat of fries and chips.

Because of the way we ate at home—a diet built primarily on vegetables, whole grains, legumes, and fruits—Rachael's diet as a whole was low in fat. I didn't want to turn fried foods into forbidden fruit, which would take on more desirability from their contraband status, so she continued to eat them away from home. These restaurant forays into fat city were infrequent enough to cause no noticeable problems for her, but her "fat taste" had developed. It was only when she was 9 years old and read something about the role of fats in causing cancer that she decided on her own to forgo them. That taught me something else: children don't need to be very old to care about their own health and want to protect it.

Because of my experiences as a parent and my background as a health writer, Dr. Attwood asked me to contribute this section to his book "from the trenches" of being a low-fat parent. We'll deal here with real-world issues, the most pressing of which has to be:

What Will We Eat?

The ideal we're striving for is to make the bulk of food choices from the "New 4 Food Groups" established by the Physicians Committee for Responsible Medicine—whole grains, vegetables, legumes (dry beans and peas), and fruits, with the optional addition of egg whites and nonfat dairy products. For most families, this need not be etched in granite. You may prefer to remain at the stage of including some lean meat or fish from time to time. Or perhaps your family is strictly vegetarian and has such a low overall fat intake that you occasionally add oil-rich nuts or avocado to your recipes. Whatever specific meals you eat, the goal is a family fat intake of around 15 percent of calories from fat.

Resist the temptation to think that when your basic fare is whole grains, vegetables, legumes, and fruit you'll be on a spartan regimen and the accolade "Delicious!" will never again be heard around your dinner table. Take heart—most of the world's people eat largely plant-based diets, and delectable vegetarian dishes abound across the globe. The plant kingdom is where the variety is, as you have read in Chapter 9 of this book.

The abundance is awesome. All the produce items and more are stocked—or can be—by any good-sized supermarket. The more unusual grains and beans (and convenience products made from them) can be purchased at a full-service natural-food store or through a food co-op.

If including such a wide variety of luxurious foods in your family menus seems cost-prohibitive, remember all the money you'll be saving when you delete many of the expensive, high-fat foods from your daily meals. Meat, cheese, butter, bakery goods, and processed foods can eat up a week's food budget yet leave the grocery cart far from full. With these eliminated or relegated to occasional use, you'll have cash to spare for the high-quality foods you'll need to grow healthy kids—for now and for their future.

You will also want to look at your cooking techniques to keep your family's fat intake low. Bake, steam, broil, or stir-fry with minimal oil; never deep-fry. "Sauté" in water, vegetable broth, defatted chicken broth, tomato juice, or wine instead of butter or oil. Replace part or all of the oil or shortening in baking with applesauce, pureed prunes, or mashed ripe banana. To avoid high-cholesterol egg yolks, substitute for each whole egg two egg whites, an ounce of low-fat tofu, half a ripe banana, or a commercial Egg Replacer powder (available at natural-food stores).

Plan to spend some time at your library or bookstore and peruse the low-fat, natural-foods cookbooks, starting with those listed in "Recommended Reading," at the end of this book. Find one or two that seem to be in keeping with your cooking style and the kinds of foods you know your family likes. (My 12-year-old sometimes plans our whole week's menus around recipes from her favorite cookbook, *The High Road to Health,* by Lindsay Wagner and Ariane Spade. It's a real confidence booster for a child to know that family and friends are eating meals she's planned or prepared.)

For more specific suggestions, look to the low-fat menus and recipes in Chapters 22 and 23. They're designed to get you well on your way toward initiating low-fat living for every family member over the age of 2.

Points to remember on foods to choose and serve:

1. The bulk of your meals will revolve around plant foods: grains (preferably whole grains), vegetables, legumes, and fruits. Reserve animal products for flavoring, occasional use, or special occasions.
2. Seek variety: a rice-and-beans rut is healthier but just as boring as a meat-and-potatoes rut. There's tremendous variety among foods that are naturally low in fat and high in complex carbohydrates. Take advantage of it.
3. Learn and use cooking and baking techniques that require little or no added oil.

Feeding Babies and Young Children

If a new baby is due at your house, or if you have an infant still on mother's milk or formula, you can start him off on a healthy lifestyle. Implement the suggestions in this book for the rest of the family, and feed your baby the same way once he reaches his second birthday.

Give mother's milk or appropriate formula exclusively for the first

12 months or so, and introduce solids slowly after that. Foods rich in iron, such as pureed peas or prunes, will be among early solids. Refrain from feeding the foods that are common allergens—cow's milk, wheat, egg white, beef, citrus fruits, shellfish, corn—until after the first birthday. Mother's milk or formula will be the primary food throughout the first year (though soft solids may be added around 6 months), and there need be no rush to wean even after that, provided your baby is not going to sleep with a bottle of formula, a practice that can damage the teeth.

Fruits, vegetables, legumes, and grains should be pureed or mashed as needed, and introduced in that order. These form the basis of an ideal diet at any age, although your family may wish to include other foods as well. In addition, the baby under 2 will be getting additional needed fat from mother's milk, formula, and some richer foods of your choice, such as avocado (mashed alone or with banana), soft-boiled egg yolk, or full-fat tofu (good pureed with a green vegetable). (For additional information on infant feeding, see *The Womanly Art of Breastfeeding* from La Leche League International, or *Pregnancy, Children, and the Vegan Diet,* by Dr. Michael Klaper, both listed in "Recommended Reading.")

Once little ones have reached age 2, they can eat in large part the way the rest of the family does. This is an excellent time to look at the family diet as a whole. In many homes, the baby has a better diet than anyone else! If a weaning infant is started on greens and fruits and plenty of fresh, natural "chew foods"—celery sticks, peeled apple slices, whole-grain teething crackers—you'll have a toddler who prefers these foods.

Unfortunately, this is the time when well-meaning relatives, friends, and bank tellers become determined to introduce your tot to cheese chunks, chocolate bars, and lollipops (low-fat but pure sugar). Practice the phrase you'll use hundreds of times: "No, thank you: she's allergic."

Tiny children are not deprived when they don't have some food they've never tasted. If you feel sorry for your child when you deny him some so-called goody, look carefully at what you're experiencing. Perhaps you're feeling sorry for yourself, since you grew up on those foods and they have emotional content for you. You as a parent have the power to create emotional content in foods for your children now. If they associate love and warmth and happy times with watermelon and corn on the cob and whole-wheat bread fresh from the oven, those will be the foods they'll like best all their lives.

Preschoolers can be easily persuaded to accept one food over another, and the wise parent carries suitable treats when away from home. The worst dietary influence on children under school age is the television set, particularly the commercials that accompany Saturday-morning cartoons. I cannot urge you strongly enough to monitor your children's television habits—the ads as well as the programs. If TV is part of your family's life-style, consider limiting your children's viewing to public television, or programs you can videotape and play back without commercials.

Alternatively, watch television with your kids and discuss the ads. Young children do not understand the concept that advertising is not undeniable truth. If the voice says, "All the kids eat Junk-e-pops," your children will feel compelled to eat them too, unless they are taught to be discriminating listeners. Consider the magnitude of this: Most adults are swayed by advertising, or corporations wouldn't spend billions of dollars on it every year. To expect children to turn a deaf ear to Madison Avenue's serenade is asking a lot.

**Points to remember for the
infancy-through-preschool years:**

1. Mother's milk or formula is the primary food for the first year and can continue beyond that time.
2. Babies under 2 need more fat than they ever will again. Meet this need with mother's milk or formula, avocado, egg yolk, and other natural, nonallergenic foods.
3. Keep little ones away from greasy food and junk food as long as possible.
4. Help your children deal with the dietary misinformation from TV commercials.

Out in the World

When children go to school, other influences intervene. Some schools still teach the original archaic "4 Food Groups," which imply that animal foods (meat and dairy products) should make up half the diet. If your children have learned something else at home, they may be confused. If there's a hot-lunch program, children believe the food served in the cafeteria must be "good" or the school, the new authority figure, wouldn't allow it. (See Chapter 17 on school lunch programs.)

If children bring bag lunches, the contents of other children's lunches are infinitely interesting. To see what is beneath the aluminum foil or inside the plastic bowl is like looking in on another family's private life—sort of a sitcom in a brown paper bag. Children are busy trying to make sense of this very big world, and somebody's else's lunch is a microcosm of that world outside their own family. Peer pressure often rears its ugly head for the first time across the lunch table. It helps if your children's low-fat lunches contain recognizable foods that don't set them apart.

Thermoses of vegetable or bean soup aren't beyond the pale; carrot and celery sticks and fresh fruit are nice "ordinary" foods, too; and low-fat cookies and puddings can be downright enviable. If you pack a sandwich, you may want to keep your homemade stone-ground whole-wheat bread at home and send a sandwich on commercial bread. If you eat meat, you can fill a sandwich with a low-fat variety such as skinned chicken. If you're further along in your dietary progression, you can use a fat-free cheese, a bean spread, or jam and a reduced-fat nut butter made by whipping the nut butter with water so a little goes further. (See the recipes in Chapter 23 for further suggestions, including Peanut-Butter Stretchers, page 232.)

The thing to remember is that any boxed lunch that looks too "different" can be threatening to another's child sense of rightness and order, causing him to say, "Ick! You eat that?" Only a child very secure within herself will be able to say, "I like my lunch. I wish your parents cared enough about you to feed you good food too." If your children are to become capable of this kind of confidence and self-assurance, they must be raised with a sense of confidence and self-assurance in general.

Other People's Opinions

When it comes to diet specifically, trust the ability of even a young child to comprehend that some foods make us well and strong and others can harm us. You can say things like, "In our home, we choose to eat the healthy foods. Some people—even good and smart people like Grandpa and your teacher—don't know what we know about food. They have a different opinion. That's okay, but we're going to eat what we know is best. Maybe someday Grandpa and Miss Smith will learn the things we know about food, just as we can learn other things from them that we don't know yet."

Criticism may still come. When my daughter was in a Mothers' Day Out day-care program at the age of 3, I always sent her lunch with a thermos of low-fat soy milk. One day I got up early and thought I'd be Supermom and make her fresh carrot juice instead. That afternoon, when I opened her lunch box to clear out the garbage (surely one of the real joys of motherhood), I found a form letter neatly folded inside. It said, "Dear Parent. We notice that your child did not have a food from each of the Four Food Groups in his lunch today. The missing food group is: ["Dairy Products" was checked.] If you do not understand the Four Food Groups, and would like counseling from our dietitian, please call us."

I was furious! The situation was all the more ludicrous in that Rachael's lunches had never included dairy products; they just *looked* as if they had. I got on the phone to every sympathetic physician and dietitian I knew. (After my 15 years as a health writer, there were quite a few.) They all faxed me letters of support. In addition, I went through my files and collected photocopies of dozens of journal articles supporting my position.

I showed up at the school the next day with so many faxes and photocopies my briefcase wouldn't shut. "I'm here to see your dietitian," I announced. She was actually a student of dietetics, working as an intern. The young woman was overwhelmed and said, "I only sent that note because some parents put cola in their kids' lunches!" I wondered how, after almost four years of training, she could mistake carrot juice for cola, but I let that go and retorted with, "Yes, and some parents put whole milk in their kids' lunches. You should be sending them notes too."

The point is, you have to be educated on nutrition in general and pediatric nutrition in particular if you are going to feed your children in a way that is still unusual in our society. It's analogous to those warnings that say, "See your doctor before you start on an exercise program." No one says, "See your doctor before you spend another day sitting on the couch rusting out."

If you choose to feed your children a lot of greasy fast food and high-fat desserts, few people expect you to know very much about nutrition. Your kids will be eating in the generally accepted way. But if you choose to feed your family a low-fat diet, particularly if you go to Stage 3 or 4 of Dr. Attwood's plan and eliminate most or all animal products from your diet, you are supposed to be a walking, talking "Nutrient Content of Foods" table.

Reading this book has already armed you with a great deal of the knowledge you need. Study Part Three, on scientific facts, until you find yourself quoting it to others. If you want still more information, refer to books listed in "Recommended Reading," at the back of this book. Remember: You may be saving your child's life just as surely as if you were diving into a lake to save him from drowning. The time you spend educating yourself will pay handsome dividends.

I have found it useful to inform the important people in our lives (doctors, teachers, neighbors, the parents of Rachael's friends) about our diet early in the relationship. (If I had done this at that Mothers' Day Out day-care program, I would have saved myself the uncomfortable situation that occurred.) Because I present our dietary choice in an informed and nonjudgmental way, I have found far more people who want to learn more about it than who want to criticize it. If someone asks a question for which I do not have an answer, I get an answer, either by consulting a professional or by doing research on my own. It's essential not to pontificate or say things like, "You should really be eating this way." Phrasing things in the first person—i.e., "I've found that eating a very low-fat diet works really well in our family"—encourages people to be interested rather than defensive.

You may also be called upon to educate your child's physician. This can be tough; doctors are supposed to be experts on diet, but most are not. If you've made a serious, independent study of nutrition, you may well be more informed and more current on the subject than the doctor is. If yours is too resistant and will not read the information you can provide him with (this book, for instance), you may need to look for another doctor. At least you need to be willing to stand up for what you know, and not be dissuaded by someone who may certainly be an expert in medicine but not necessarily in nutrition.

Points to remember for the school-age years:

1. Teach your children the importance of a low-fat diet. Let them know that, though some people have different ideas, "This is what we do in our family."
2. Work with your child's school to develop an appropriate hot-lunch program. If you pack a lunch for your child, make it look "normal" to spare your child unnecessary taunting.
3. Educate yourself about low-fat nutrition and what children need to grow into healthy adults. Have confidence in your educated conclusions.
4. Discuss your child's dietary requirements with the teacher at the beginning of the year. Look for a pediatrician who is knowledgeable about low-fat diets for children, or willing to research the subject.

Eating Extremes

Most childen have some peculiarities about food. They don't like certain tastes, textures, or colors. They suddenly won't eat something they liked last week, because this week it's touching another food on the plate. Or they'll want one food over and over for weeks on end. It takes courage to add the variable of a low-fat diet into all this, but it's important enough to be brave and go forward.

The two eating extremes that worry parents most concern the child who overeats and is overweight, and the finicky eater who seems to subsist like a human begonia on the rays from the sun. These are both areas of interest to me, since I was an overweight child and I gave birth to a picky eater.

Low-fat dining can be a real boon to the overweight youngster, because with it she can still eat heartily and feel full. She can have seconds and desserts and low-fat substitutes for high-fat treats, minimizing the feelings of deprivation and isolation inherent in conventional "dieting"—an approach which seldom results in truly "losing" pounds, only misplacing them for a while.

Childhood obesity is dangerous, but putting a child "on a diet" is far more so. At worst, it can lead to a host of stubborn eating disorders—even life-threatening anorexia nervosa. At best, repeated diet failures lead to eroded self-esteem and a more deeply entrenched state of overweight or obesity. If the chubby child is the only one in the family on a low-fat regimen, it's no better psychologically than any "diet." When the entire family eats in this healthy way, however, the overweight child is not singled out. His weight loss is a natural outcome—like Dad's lower cholesterol level, and his big sister's clearer complexion.

Regular physical activity is important too, but sports and rugged exercise can be torture for the overweight girl or boy. Instead, sensitively look into this child's unique interests. Would she like to walk with you in the evenings after dinner to get some one-on-one talking time? Has she ever expressed an interest in some physical activity, such as skating or horseback riding? Could you arrange to include these in her week? Going slowly and gently pays great dividends. (The first activity may not be the one that becomes a longtime interest. In other words, sign up for half a dozen riding lessons; don't buy the horse.)

Finally, children with weight issues are often using food to help them deal with the stresses of life. It can be difficult for a parent to admit that his or her child has any emotional difficulties, but instead of wasting time on denial, guilt, and blame, get your child the help she needs—professional counseling if necessary. And remember every day to let your overweight child know that she is loved *unconditionally*. She needs to know that you approve of her just the way she is. A solid sense of self-worth is the best hedge against compulsive eating and other eating disorders.

On the other hand, you may have a child who is markedly uninterested in food. Curtailing any nutrients—even artery-clogging saturated fat—in an already limited intake is not always an easy step to take. Nevertheless, children don't starve themselves to death. Look at your picky eater's actual food intake and determine what he is really consuming. It is probably more than you think. When the foods you keep in your fridge and cupboards are for the most part whole, healthful, low-fat, and minimally processed, your child can make his choices, however choosy he is, from the best possible foods.

My daughter was inordinately finicky during all her early-elementary years, but when I subjected her 10-item diet of choice to computer analysis, it turned out to be nutritionally complete. Rachael chose to eat little besides pastas, potatoes, tofu, brown rice, wheat bread, plums, oranges, raw carrots, artichokes, and—of all things!—seaweed. I also saw that she drank fortified soy milk and got a children's multivitamin-and-mineral supplement each day. She survived and grew normally. I survived too, and I learned that the finicky period invariably passes, like all of childhood's stages. (And isn't it bizarre that, once a trying stage has been gone for a while, we can remember it as rather quaint?)

If you have a picky eater, introducing a low-fat dietary program may actually help the situation, since natural, high-complex-carbohydrate foods are *simple*. Complicated dishes are the *bête noire* of most finicky kids. Making food attractive and appealing is also important in encouraging the undereager eater, and remember that all children have exceptionally sensitive taste buds—the firehouse chili or the piquant curry dish your guests rave about is not for your 7-year-old.

Also, keep foods familiar. If your child has been eating hamburgers, test several of the frozen vegetarian burgers at your natural-food store and learn to make some low-fat, meatless burgers yourself. The bun, the ketchup, the pickle, and the rest are a bigger part of the burger mystique than the hamburger itself anyway. Today there are also low-fat and fat-free versions of hot dogs, cookies, ice "cream," cheese—all the picky eaters' favorite treats. These are seldom nutritional gold mines, but including some of them in your menus can make an easier transition to low-fat meals.

The most difficult part of dealing with reluctant little diners is resisting the urge to nag. The experienced mothers I've consulted on this all agree: Beyond inviting these children at least to taste new foods, leave them alone. They'll come around. Meanwhile, keep mealtime light and happy for everyone. Complaints and criticisms can wait for a more appropriate setting.

If your child is actually underweight, finicky eater or not, starting a low-fat regimen may seem foolhardy. You don't want him to disappear! But the American idea of average weight is, when viewed from a worldwide perspective, on the high side. If your child feels good about himself and your pediatrician assures you that he is healthy, you can safely cut the fat in family meals and see if your child's natural hunger drive will make up for less fat with more food.

If this doesn't happen, focus on the more dense carbohydrate foods (flour products like bread and pasta are among them), and add the concentrated sweets and fats from the plant kingdom. Trail mix is no friendly snack for the weight watcher, but it's fine for a lean, active young person on a largely complex-carbohydrate diet. Dried fruits, avocado, soy products such as tempeh and full-fat tofu, nuts, nut butters, sunflower and pumpkin seeds, olives, and salad dressings containing cold-pressed olive or canola oil can add substantial calories in a reasonable manner.

Points to remember for over- and undereager eaters:

1. Refrain from singling out the overweight child, and make low-fat eating and healthful activity the family norm.

2. If you think your child eats for emotional reasons, make building her self-esteem your top priority. Seek professional help if needed.

3. Provide your finicky eater with whole, healthful, simple foods. Do your best to avoid nagging.

4. If your thin child is healthy, don't try too hard to "fatten him up." Allow him access to an ample, low-fat diet with plenty of bread and pasta and supplement with rich plant foods such as dried fruit and nuts.

The Food-Smart Family

Regardless of their unique dietary styles, all our children need to be educated about the importance of good nutrition. Once this is a natural part of their world view, it's theirs forever, particularly during the teen years, when eating well is vital but seldom practiced. The lion's share of this education is not formally taught; it's absorbed as if by osmosis through habitual patterning, what is being etched into their psyches day after day as "normal."

Let me prove it. "Balanced meal." Quick—what popped into your mind? I'd bet money that, instead of the kind of eating you've learned about in this book or from other dietary data you've gleaned as an adult, your picture of a so-called balanced meal is the sort of dinner you ate when you were growing up.

I've been a vegetarian for 25 years, a fat-conscious vegetarian for 10, and yet when I hear "balanced meal," my immediate mental response is to see one of the blue-and-white china "everyday plates" of my childhood with a piece of meat loaf or fried chicken and mashed potatoes with brown gravy. On the side are a little bowl of iceberg-lettuce salad drenched in Italian dressing, a glass of whole milk, and a piece of apple pie, preferably à la mode.

I've consciously changed the way I eat, but my psyche is still back at fried chicken and apple pie, because I was raised that way. Our children can receive healthier patterning, and even when they're making their own food choices, a great deal of that will stick. We can provide them with what the behavior-modification people call "state-conditioned training": in the state of having to make food choices, they're conditioned to make healthy ones.

Making the Switch

In the best of all possible worlds, you'd be reading this book as a young adult contemplating the sort of diet that would be best for your children when you have them a few years from now. Your potential spouse would have done the same preparation and be in solid agreement with you on this, and you would know from the start how you are going to feed your family.

It's far more likely, however, that you already have children who are accustomed to eating in a different way from the one suggested in this book. Your little kids may be great fans of fast-food eateries, with their playgrounds and bright, boxed meals for children. Your teenagers may seem to subsist on hamburgers and pizza alone yet somehow miraculously avoid the deficiency diseases you (and they) learned about in biology class.

The amount of control you have over what your children eat decreases exponentially as they get older, but even a 2-year-old has definite ideas about what he will and will not eat. It's crucial that mealtimes be pleasant, that the low-fat foods you prepare be tasty and attractive, and that you approach this new way of eating with a spirit of adventure.

If you want your children to go along with a dietary change, it must be fun. Grow a garden. Plant a fruit tree. Shop at farmers' markets and roadside produce stands in season. Celebrate the summer's first peaches, the fall's bright pumpkins, and traditional holiday dishes you can prepare in low-fat form. Plan your menus for color and texture and nuances in flavor. Let your children prepare fun, low-fat foods such as those in the recipes in Chapter 23.

Let your new way of eating enhance rather than detract from your joy of living. Don't stop baking cookies: learn from the recipes that follow and from other sources how to bake low-fat cookies that rate high on the yummy scale. If holidays are major feasts at your house, let them be so. Simply alter a few of the courses and the recipes so they're healthy feasts.

Visit ethnic restaurants for ideas on exotic fare that may contain far less saturated fat and total fat than many familiar specialties. Look into joining a food co-op or a buying club that can enable you to purchase natural foods at a substantial discount and will connect you with other families trying to eat healthfully. If your child makes a friend who eats similarly, it can be a real boon to her healthy eating efforts.

The Disagreeing Spouse

You may also run into the situation of wanting very much to cut the fat in your family's meals but finding your husband or wife adamantly opposed to it. Earlier in this essay, I suggested that you need to become something of a nutrition expert to communicate with teachers, physicians, and friends. Now I'm suggesting that you become skilled in diplomacy to introduce a new way of eating in your own home.

The fact is, human beings do not like change, especially when the change involves something as basic as how we eat. Even young children identify themselves by their food choices: "My name is Meg and I'm five years old and I have a dog and I liked grilled-cheese sandwiches and ice cream with chocolate sauce." Change imposed from the outside is much harder to take than self-generated change. That's where your diplomacy will come in. If your spouse and children *want* to eat healthfully now to avoid problems later, you'll have allies in your efforts.

Getting your partner on your side may be the single most important thing you can do in your attempt to change your children's diet. When one parent wants to make a change and the other does not, the children tend to side with the one who's for maintaining the status quo. When both parents are committed to something that affects the entire family, however, the children tend to follow. (Teens, of course, would lose face dreadfully if they felt they were following their parents, but even they will be watching and learning.)

Share this book with your significant other. Every person in America who hasn't been unconscious since the mid-1980s knows that eating less fat is critical in our effort to stem the tide of degenerative disease. Many adults have made sweeping changes in their food choices, but others have resisted. Either way, most of us have not realized the importance of a low-fat diet for our children. Since parents are somehow programmed by nature to do for their offspring what is too much effort to do for themselves, getting this information to your husband or wife could be the turning point in making low-fat eating a family affair.

If you do not have the support of your partner, rest assured that you're not alone. Probably the number-one question I'm asked when I speak to groups is how to deal with a recalcitrant spouse! My answer is always: "Make whatever subtle but important changes you can, and keep the overall picture in mind." Your children are what they eat, but they're a lot more than that as well. Their health also depends on exercise, adequate rest and sleep, fresh air, and more subtle elements such as feeling loved and worthy. I am convinced that having a stable family life without parental discord over a daily issue like "What's for dinner?" is more significant than whether a child's diet contains 15 percent of calories from fat or 25 during the transitional stages.

Of course, if your family has been eating the standard U.S. diet, with 40 percent of its calories in the form of fat, even getting to 25 is going to take some doing. This can, however, be done gradually—particularly if you meet with a great deal of resistance from your partner. If you're not the regular cook in the family, get yourself a chef's apron and take over dinner duties more often.

In the traditional situation, in which the woman cooks most of the time, she's usually thrilled to eat something someone else has prepared. In a high percentage of the cases that I run into, however, it is the woman who wants to cut dietary fat while the man believes that thick cuts of beef are physiological necessities for testosterone production. Real men eat red meat, right? Unfortunately, that kind of real man is often setting himself up for a very real massive coronary, as well as passing on a deadly myth to his children.

Small Changes

Negotiation and education can work wonders in this situation. If you can share what you learn with your partner without force-feeding the information, his own intelligence, sense of self-preservation, and love for his children may be enough to change his mind. And you can always make small dietary changes that are barely perceptible but can nevertheless result in an appreciable decrease in total fat intake. Try these to start with:

1. Make omelettes using 2 egg whites for each whole egg.
2. Use meat as part of a larger dish rather than the center of the meal—a stir-fry with lots of vegetables and some chicken, chili with plenty of beans and less ground beef, hearty lentil and split-pea and potato soups with a bit of meat for flavoring.
3. Bone up on ethnic cooking—entrées of Indian, Italian, Mexican, or Chinese derivation are often based on grains, beans, and vegetables that are virtually fat-free.
4. Experiment with low-oil and no-oil salad dressings and only serve the ones that really taste rich and good.
5. Change dessert recipes to satisfy all the sweet teeth at your house without the fat that usually accompanies pastries and goodies. For example, make apple crisp instead of apple pie (the crust is full of fat), serve sorbet or nonfat frozen yogurt instead of ice cream, make an angel-food cake instead of one rich in fat and cholesterol.
6. Stock up on low-fat snacks. In addition to fresh fruit and crudités—the healthiest snacks of all—look to pretzels, air-popped corn and—for special treats—the many low-fat cookies and chips now available commercially. (My daughter and her friends love Barbecue Mini Rice Cakes from Hain and the baked potato chips called Popsters from American Grains.)
7. Use the recipes in this book, and consult "Recommended Reading" for additional reading material and cookbooks.
8. If your situation requires serving meat-centered dinners much of the time, do your best to see that your children's breakfasts,

lunches, and snacks are consistently low in fat. Remember: it's the overall picture that counts. You're not imposing some rigid "diet"; you're building healthy habits your sons and daughters will take with them into adulthood.

Whatever you do, be gentle with yourself and those around you. Family life is never easy, and in today's world it can be fraught with complications. You may be a working, single parent who greatly appreciates fast-food restaurants for making your life a little easier. Don't try to give up fast food entirely; just choose places with salad bars, pasta, and baked potatoes as often as you can. Your children may not live with you full-time, and your influence on what they eat at the home of their other parent may be minimal or nonexistent. Feed your children as well as you know how when they're with you, and trust the integrity of their strong, young bodies to deal with what they're fed elsewhere.

You may be juggling all sorts of conflicting needs—an overweight child, an underweight child, a son who's allergic to dairy products, a daughter who's allergic to wheat, preschoolers who need to be in bed by 7:00 and a spouse who doesn't get home for dinner until 8:00. Calm down. Slow down. Take a deep breath and make those tiny changes one at a time. Use Dr. Attwood's stages to guide your progress.

Allow your family's eating pattern to evolve into one that is low in fat and high in complex carbohydrates, one in which animal foods are downplayed (or perhaps even eliminated) and whole grains, beans, vegetables, and fruit are standard fare. And at whatever stage you are in your dietary advancement, stir some love in with whatever you've got on the stove. It may sound simplistic, but think about it: food from caring cooks *tastes better,* and I have a hunch that love-seasoned meals nourish us in a very special way.

Points to remember for a food-smart family:

1. Educate your children about healthy low-fat food both with your words and, more important, with the foods you keep on hand and the meals you serve.

2. Make the changes interesting, delicious, and fun. Invite your children to help with shopping and cooking, even though this "help" can make the process more time-consuming.

3. Enlist your spouse's support. Share this book with him or her.

4. If your partner is not enthusiastic about a low-fat diet, make small, gradual changes. Do your best to keep family harmony and good nutrition in balance. (I realize that in some households this can be a tall order.)

5. Lighten up on yourself as you switch your family to a lighter diet. Be good to yourself, so you have energy left for preparing meals with caring and love. Your aim is not dietary perfection but continual improvement and a happy, healthy family.

Chapter 22

Suggested Menus

BY VICTORIA MORAN

*A*lways take menus with a grain of salt—whether you keep to a low-sodium diet or not! A new way of eating sticks only when it reflects your family's preferences and life-style, your ethnic background, your budget, and the foods that are readily available where you live. When you make your own menus, plan them around the seasons: hot cereals and steaming soups in the winter, chilled fruit dishes and salads in the summer. (Enjoy pungent, spicy foods in warm weather as well: these "hot" foods tend to cool the body—witness their popularity in the lands of eternal summer, such as India and Mexico.)

Cooking for children—like every other aspect of dealing with them—takes a tremendous amount of patience. Almost every unfamiliar dish is likely to be greeted by a resounding "Yuk!" Be persistent. Children are almost infinitely flexible. One of the nicest things about natural, low-fat dining is that there is so much to choose from—dozens of beans and grains, hundreds of vegetables and fruits—that eating this way need never be boring. In addition, no one food is required for a healthy diet. If your child doesn't like spinach or raisins or pinto beans, it doesn't matter; there are plenty of other foods with the same nutrients.

Take what you like from these sample menus, designed to meet or approach the Stage 4 guidelines of Dr. Attwood's program. Let your children help you plan additional menus. After all, they know what they like. (Note: The recipes for dishes in the menus marked with asterisks may be found in the recipe section, in Chapter 23.)

Breakfasts

Low-fat breakfasts with customary components generally include grains, fruits and juices, and nonfat milk or a low-fat, nondairy milk substitute fortified with calcium and vitamin D. The following breakfasts fit this pattern, but use your imagination: many children prefer to eat nontraditional breakfasts. You may even get by from time to time with something exotic, like Japanese-inspired rice and vegetables.

- Oatmeal with blueberries and sliced peaches, nonfat or soy milk
- Banana pancakes* and real maple syrup, nonfat or soy milk
- Fresh orange juice, low-fat granola,* or whole-grain boxed cereal with nonfat or soy milk
- Broiled grapefruit with honey, whole-grain toast with a peanut-butter stretcher* and all-fruit jam, cocoa- or carob-flavored nonfat or soy milk
- Tomato juice, baked beans on toast, nonfat or soy milk
- Nonfat or soy yogurt with fresh strawberries, oat-bran muffins with all-fruit jam, apple juice
- Tropical fruit salad—oranges, pineapple, kiwi, mango—with nonfat cottage cheese, applesauce muffins,* nonfat or soy milk
- Smoothie: nonfat or soy milk or yogurt, ripe banana (fresh or peeled and frozen overnight), frozen strawberries, honey to taste (also see Strawberry-Banana Fruit Shake* in recipe section)
- Scrambled fat-reduced tofu (the easiest way to scramble tofu is with the ready-made commercial product Tofu Scrambler, from Fantastic Foods), whole-grain toast with all-fruit jam, calcium-fortified orange juice

- Omelette, substituting 2 egg whites for each whole egg, oven fries,* stewed apples, nonfat or soy milk
- Grape juice, "Danish" made from nonfat cottage cheese sweetened with honey, vanilla, and cinnamon spread on slices of bread and baked in toaster oven, nonfat or soy milk
- Cranberry juice, cinnamon-raisin bagel with low-fat dairy or soy cream cheese, nonfat or soy milk

Lunches

For summers, Saturdays, and the lunch box, soups, salads, and sandwiches are what we're used to. These can adapt well to a low-fat diet, even at Stage 4. Make lunches colorful, tasty, and hearty. When you pack a lunch for kids to take to school, frequently include a healthy treat, and every so often tuck in a tiny toy or a special note ("Today after school we'll go to the park"). Save unusual food for your kids to sample at home: seaweed may have much to recommend it, but not in the school cafeteria.

- Raw vegetables and fat-free chips with hummus* (garbanzo dip), pasta salad,* strawberry nonfat or soy yogurt, fresh lemonade
- Barbecued bean sandwich (coarsely puree a can of drained beans with ⅛ to ¼ cup of barbecue sauce to make a spread), tossed salad with veggie salad dressing,* gingerbread cookies,* nonfat or soy milk
- Lentil soup, fat-free crackers, carrot and celery sticks, chocolate-chip cranberry cookies,* nonfat or soy milk
- Baked beans, corn bread,* potato salad,* apple, nonfat or soy milk
- Salad in a pita (stuff a pita pocket with leaf lettuce, grated carrot, sprouts, garbanzos, and a sauce of seasoned nonfat yogurt), split-pea soup, low-fat chocolate pudding (Dream Pudding from Imagine Foods is fat-free and comes ready to eat in individual-serving sizes, at natural-food stores)
- Burritos (see recipe for "refried" beans*), low-fat corn chips and

raw-veggie platter with salsa, frozen fruit-juice pops, nonfat or soy milk

- Veggie-burger (see page 117, "Meat Substitutes") on whole-grain burger rolls, oven fries,* carrot and celery sticks, banana "ice cream,"* natural soda made from fruit juice and sparkling water
- "Sunny sandwich" (add ground raw hulled sunflower seeds to plain nonfat yogurt and season to taste—a bit of chili powder perks it up for those who like spice), potato-corn chowder,* broccoli and cauliflower florets, big Medjool dates, apple juice
- Fat-free cheese slices with apple and pear, fat-free crackers and rice cakes, natural soda
- Peanut-butter-stretcher* sandwich with lettuce and all-fruit jam, red and green pepper slices, "mud" cookies,* nonfat or soy milk
- Vegetarian chili,* fat-free saltines, salsa or pico de gallo, pine-apple upside-down cake,* nonfat or soy milk
- Lean meat or meatlike sandwich (sliced chicken with the skin removed or fat-free meatless slices like Smart Deli Thin Slices from Lightlife Foods), tomato-vegetable soup,* banana, carob- or cocoa-flavored soy milk or rice beverage

Dinners

The traditional picture of a formal dinner with the whole family around the table sharing stories of their day is little more than folk-lore in many modern households. I think it's important enough to try to salvage, no matter how much energy it takes.

For many busy children (and adults), dinner is the only meal with a ghost of a chance of being consumed in a leisurely fashion. It's the meal that can pack concentrated nutrition, and the one that can be seriously low in fat, without compromising for lunch-box limitations or school lunch shortfalls. This is also the time when a cook with the slightest hint of creativity can really shine.

- Pasta with marinara sauce, Italian bread, three-bean salad with oil-free vinaigrette, raspberry sorbet, sparkling red grape juice
- Shepherd's pie (use your favorite vegetables and a fluffy potato crust), salad or leaf lettuce and fresh tomatoes with seasoned rice vinegar, biscuits, apple crisp,* nonfat or soy milk
- Stir-fried vegetables with fat-reduced tofu or white meat of chicken (if you need more moisture in a stir-fry, add vegetable broth instead of extra oil), steamed rice, miso-noodle soup, carrot-raisin salad (use nonfat mayonnaise or nonfat yogurt), or fresh fruit platter, hot or iced herbal tea
- Eggplant lasagna,* steamed kale, salad with creamy vinaigrette (add fat-reduced tofu or cottage cheese to your favorite oil-free vinaigrette and blend), fruit basket, chocolate-brownie cake,* hot or iced herbal tea
- Lentil loaf with chunky tomato sauce, mashed potatoes, peas and carrots, frozen yogurt or fat-free nondairy dessert, nonfat or soy milk
- Black beans and rice, spinach salad with nonfat vinaigrette dressing, steamed or baked yams, nonfat or soy milk
- Rice and dal (lentils or split peas with turmeric and garam masala—go easy on the spice for small children), steamed string beans, banana-oat muffins,* fresh-fruit gelatin (if you prefer vegetarian gelatin, use agar flakes from the natural-food store), nonfat or soy milk
- Vegetable Pizza,* salad of romaine, cauliflorets, Italian plum tomatoes, and garbanzos, commercial fat-free cookies, nonfat or soy milk
- Split-pea soup, salad of baby greens with nonfat dessing, bran muffins, fruit compote, natural soda
- Baked haddock or grilled, marinated tofu (fat-reduced), sweet-and-sour red cabbage, corn on the cob, sliced apples and pears, fresh fruit or vegetable juice
- Black-eyed peas, spaghetti squash, mixed green salad with oil-free vinaigrette, low-fat rice pudding, nonfat or soy milk

Chapter 23

Children-Tested Recipes

BY SONNET PIERCE

Breakfast

Banana "Ice Cream"

Banana Pancakes

Fruit-Juice Smoothies and
Shakes

Low-Fat Granola

Lunch

Hummus

Pasta Salad

Peanut-Butter Stretchers

Potato Salad

Tomato-Vegetable Soup

Veggie Salad Dressing

Supper

Oven Fries

Potato-Corn Chowder

"Refried" Beans

Super-Saucy Eggplant Lasagna

Vegetable Pizza

Vegetarian Chili

Desserts and Breads

Apple Crisp

Applesauce Muffins

Banana-Oat Muffins

Chocolate-Brownie Cake

Chocolate-Chip
Cranberry Cookies

Corn Bread

Gingerbread Cookies

"Mud" Cookies

Introduction

This section contains recipes that I have developed while experimenting with low-fat and vegetarian cooking. Many of these recipes are healthy versions of traditional foods, such as pizza, cookies, and ice cream. If we prepare low-fat versions of foods that children are familiar with, it is much easier for them (and us) to make the transition between a high-fat diet and a low-fat one. When you prepare these recipes yourself, you will discover that it is possible to eliminate meat, eggs, dairy products, and fat from your diet without sacrificing flavor.

In these recipes, I have tried to use ingredients that are easy to find. Most of them can be bought at your local grocery store, but a few of the items will have to be purchased at a natural-food store.

Breakfast

BANANA "ICE CREAM"

*I was excited when I came across this idea, and after
some experimenting I came up with these variations.
I eat this "ice cream" for breakfast with granola
and for dessert on hot evenings.*

2 bananas
1 tablespoon fruit juice *or*
    skim milk

1. Peel the bananas, break them into pieces, and freeze them in a plastic container for 12 hours, or until they are hard. (I like to keep a container of bananas in the freezer so that I have them when I feel like having "ice cream.")
2. Remove bananas from freezer and let them sit out at room temperature for 15 minutes, or until they start to soften.

3. In a food processor, with a metal blade, process bananas until they are broken up into small pieces. Add the juice and process until smooth. Serve immediately.

For 1 serving:

WITH JUICE	WITH SKIM MILK
Per serving:	*Per serving:*
217 calories	215 calories
2.5 gm protein	2.9 gm protein
1.1 gm fat	1.1 gm fat
0.4 gm sat. fat	0.4 gm sat. fat
0.0 mg cholesterol	0.3 mg cholesterol

Variations:

BLUEBERRY "ICE CREAM"
 1 frozen banana
 ½ cup frozen blueberries
 1 tablespoon fruit juice *or*
    skim milk

Follow directions for Banana "Ice Cream," but replace 1 of the bananas with the blueberries.

WITH JUICE	WITH SKIM MILK
Per serving:	*Per serving:*
152 calories	151 calories
1.8 gm protein	2.2 gm protein
0.8 gm fat	0.9 gm fat
0.2 gm sat. fat	0.2 gm sat. fat
0.0 mg cholesterol	0.3 mg cholesterol

STRAWBERRY "ICE CREAM"

1 frozen banana
⅔ cup frozen strawberries
 (10 strawberries)

1 tablespoon fruit juice *or*
 skim milk

Follow directions for Banana "Ice Cream," but replace 1 of the bananas with the strawberries.

WITH JUICE	WITH SKIM MILK
Per serving:	*Per serving:*
275 calories	273 calories
2.2 gm protein	2.6 gm protein
0.8 gm fat	0.8 gm fat
0.2 gm sat. fat	0.2 gm sat. fat
0.0 mg cholesterol	0.3 mg cholesterol

Additional Variations: Use frozen mangoes, peaches, blackberries, or raspberries. Be creative!

BANANA PANCAKES

*After many experiments I came up with this pancake
recipe that contains no oil or eggs. They are delicious and
much more filling than the pancakes made from a mix.*

¾ cup whole-wheat flour
½ cup all-purpose white flour
¼ cup cornmeal
1 tablespoon baking powder
½ teaspoon salt
½ cup mashed banana

1½ cups water
⅛ teaspoon lemon extract
 (optional)
1 tablespoon powdered Egg
 Replacer*
3 tablespoons water

* Egg Replacer is a fat-free powder egg substitute made by Energy Foods that can be found at natural-food stores.

1. With a wire whisk, mix together flours, cornmeal, baking powder, and salt.
2. Mix together banana, water, and flavoring (if used) in a separate bowl.
3. Preheat a griddle or a large skillet (nonstick or lightly oiled).
4. With an electric mixer on high speed, beat the Egg Replacer with the water for 2 minutes (Egg Replacer will get foamy and begin to get stiff).
5. Stir together Egg Replacer and banana mixture.
6. Whisk together wet and dry mixtures until thoroughly combined. Don't worry about lumps.
7. When a few drops of water sprinkled on the griddle bead up and roll off, the griddle is ready.
8. Use ¼ cup of batter for each pancake. Cook the pancakes for 1½–2 minutes on the hot griddle, or until the bottoms are lightly browned. Flip pancakes and cook another ½–1 minute, or until the bottoms are set and freckled. Serve hot with syrup, jam, or fruit.

For 12 4-inch pancakes (4 servings):

Per serving (3 pancakes):
199 calories / 7.0 gm protein / 0.9 gm fat / 0.2 gm sat. fat / 0.0 mg cholesterol

FRUIT-JUICE SMOOTHIES AND SHAKES

*By using different fruit juices and fresh or
frozen fruit, you can make endless varieties
of delicious fruit shakes with frozen bananas
and smoothies with unfrozen bananas.*

BASIC BANANA SMOOTHIE:

1 banana
1 cup fruit juice (orange juice,
    pineapple juice, cranberry-
    juice cocktail, grape juice,
    or your favorite fruit juice)

Combine ingredients in a blender and blend on high speed until smooth.

For one serving:

Per serving:
217 calories / 2.9 gm protein / 0.7 gm fat / 0.2 gm sat. fat /
0.0 mg cholesterol

BANANA-BERRY SMOOTHIE:

1 cup fruit juice
1 banana
¼ cup berries

Follow directions for Basic Banana Smoothie.

For one serving:

Per serving:
228 calories / 3.1 gm protein / 0.8 gm fat / 0.2 gm sat. fat /
0.0 mg cholesterol

STRAWBERRY-BANANA FRUIT SHAKE:

1 cup orange juice
1 frozen banana*
6 to 8 frozen strawberries

Follow directions for Basic Banana Smoothie.

For one serving:

Per serving:
318 calories / 3.4 gm protein / 0.8 gm fat / 0.2 gm sat. fat /
0.0 mg cholesterol

BERRY SHAKE:

1 cup cranberry-juice cocktail
1 frozen banana*
¼ cup frozen blueberries

Follow directions for Basic Banana Smoothie.

For one serving:

Per serving:
296 calories / 1.5 gm protein / 1.0 gm fat / 0.3 gm sat. fat /
0.0 mg cholesterol

* To freeze bananas: peel, break into pieces, and freeze in an airtight container.

LOW-FAT GRANOLA

*This sweet, crunchy granola is great as
a breakfast cereal. It is also good as a topping
over fresh fruit or Banana "Ice Cream."*

9 cups rolled oats
½ cup wheat bran
¼ cup nuts *or* seeds (such as
   slivered almonds,
   chopped walnuts, or
   sunflower seeds)
3 teaspoons cinnamon

½ teaspoon nutmeg
1¼ cup honey
¼ 6-ounce can frozen grape-
   juice concentrate, thawed
1 cup dried fruit (such as
   raisins, apples, apricots,
   or dates)

1. In a large bowl, mix together the oats, wheat bran, nuts, cinnamon, and nutmeg.
2. In a small bowl, beat together honey and grape-juice concentrate.
3. Thoroughly mix together wet and dry mixtures.
4. Spread mixture on baking sheets that have been lightly oiled or sprayed with cooking spray. (Be sure to use baking sheets that have sides.)
5. Bake at 350 degrees F. for approximately 20 minutes, stirring often to avoid burning, until light to medium brown. Mixture may seem moist, but it will dry as it cools.
6. When mixture is cool, add dried fruit, and store in airtight containers.

For 20 ½-cup servings:

Per serving:
245 calories / 6.6 gm protein / 3.4 gm fat / 0.5 gm sat. fat /
0.0 mg cholesterol

Lunch

HUMMUS

Hummus, a spread made from chick-peas (garbanzo beans),
is usually served cold on pita bread.

2 cups cooked or canned
    chick-peas (garbanzo
    beans)
2 tablespoons lemon juice
2 tablespoons cooking liquid
    from chick-peas

1 teaspoon granulated garlic
2 teaspoons chopped fresh
    parsley
¼–½ teaspoon salt (to taste)

1. In a food processor, with a metal blade, process all ingredients until smooth.
2. Serve on pita bread with lettuce, cucumbers, sprouts, chopped tomatoes, or any of your favorite vegetables.

For 4 ½-cup servings:

Per serving:
139 calories / 7.4 gm protein / 2.2 gm fat / 0.2 gm sat. fat / 0.0 mg cholesterol

PASTA SALAD

This is a colorful salad, especially when vegetable-semolina (multicolored) pasta is used. For a different twist, use your favorite in-season vegetables in this salad.*

3 cups dry pasta, cooked, drained, and rinsed with cold water
1 15-ounce can tomato sauce (Hunt's Natural, no salt added)
1 tablespoon cornstarch
1 teaspoon dried oregano
1 teaspoon dried basil

2 cups finely chopped carrots
5 scallions (green onions), finely chopped
1 10-ounce package frozen corn, thawed (1½ cups corn kernels)
4 ounces fresh or canned mushrooms, drained
salt and pepper to taste

1. In a small saucepan, whisk together tomato sauce, cornstarch, oregano, and basil.
2. Bring tomato-sauce mixture to a boil, whisking constantly, and simmer for a couple of minutes or until thickened. Let cool.
3. In a medium-sized bowl, mix together the cooked pasta and the vegetables.
4. Pour the tomato sauce over the pasta-vegetable mixture and add salt and pepper to taste. Store in the refrigerator until ready to serve.

For 7 servings:

Per serving:
295 calories / 10.2 gm protein / 1.3 gm fat / 0.2 gm sat. fat / 0.0 mg cholesterol

* Some vegetables that are good additions to this salad are tomatoes, grated zucchini, bell peppers, celery, and green peas. You can also add fresh basil or parsley.

PEANUT-BUTTER STRETCHERS

*Peanut butter is a high-fat food, but by
stretching it with bananas or sweet potatoes,
you can enjoy the peanut flavor without as much fat.*

STRETCHER #1:
2 tablespoons mashed banana
1 teaspoon peanut butter

Mix together the banana and peanut butter, and use it in place of
plain peanut butter on a sandwich.

For one serving:

Per serving:
57 calories / 1.6 gm protein / 2.8 gm fat / 0.6 gm sat. fat /
0.0 mg cholesterol

STRETCHER #2:
2 tablespoons cooked and
    mashed sweet potato
1 teaspoon peanut butter
1 teaspoon honey

Mix together all the ingredients and serve in place of plain peanut
butter on a sandwich.

For one serving:

Per serving:
86 calories / 1.9 gm protein / 2.7 gm fat / 0.5 gm sat. fat /
0.0 mg cholesterol

POTATO SALAD

*Potato salad is usually high in fat, because it has
a sauce that contains mayonnaise. The sauce for this potato
salad uses cornstarch instead, in an unexpected way.*

10 medium unpeeled potatoes,
    boiled, cooled, and cut
    into cubes (8 cups
    cooked)
3 tablespoons cornstarch
1 cup cold water
    juice of 1 small lemon
    (¼ cup)
2 teaspoons salt (or to taste)
½ teaspoon black pepper
    (or to taste)
1 teaspoon basil

1 tablespoon chopped fresh
    parsley
2–3 tablespoons prepared
    mustard
1 tablespoon honey
1 cup grated carrot
1 cup frozen green peas,
    thawed
½ cup finely chopped celery
⅓ cup finely chopped onion
½ cup chopped pickles *or*
    pickle relish

1. In a small saucepan, whisk together cornstarch and water and
   bring to a boil over high heat, stirring constantly, until thickened.
   Remove from heat and cool.
2. Mix lemon juice, salt, pepper, basil, parsley, mustard, and honey
   into the cornstarch mixture.
3. In a large bowl, combine the potatoes, carrot, peas, celery, onion, and pickle.
4. Pour sauce over the potatoes and vegetables, and mix well. Ad-
   just seasoning to taste.

Note: My main purpose with this recipe is to give you the basic idea
of using cornstarch-thickened water in place of mayonnaise. I encourage you to change your favorite potato-salad recipe using this
technique.

For 10 servings:

Per serving:
146 calories / 3.4 gm protein / 0.4 gm fat / 0.1 gm sat. fat / 0.0 mg cholesterol

===

TOMATO-VEGETABLE SOUP

This is a good soup to put in a thermos for lunch.

2 teaspoons oil
2 cups chopped onion
2 cups chopped celery
2 cups chopped carrot
4 cups chopped potatoes
1 46-fluid-ounce can
    tomato juice
1 teaspoon each dried
    oregano, basil, and thyme

1 tablespoon dried parsley
1 cup corn kernels (fresh,
    frozen, or canned)
1 tablespoon brown sugar
    (optional)
    salt and pepper

1. In a 6-quart pot, heat oil over high heat.
2. Sauté the onion in the oil for 1 minute.
3. Stir in the celery and carrots and sauté 2 minutes more.
4. Add the potatoes and cook for 5 minutes more, stirring often.
5. Stir in the tomato juice and herbs.
6. Bring to a boil, and simmer for 25 minutes, or until vegetables are tender.
7. Add the corn, sugar (if desired), and salt and pepper to taste.
8. Heat well.

For 6 main-course servings:

Per serving:
223 calories / 5.8 gm protein / 2.3 gm fat / 0.4 gm sat. fat /
0.0 mg cholesterol

VEGGIE SALAD DRESSING

*This fat-free salad dressing
is good on green salads.*

8 ounces tomato sauce
3 tablespoons seasoned rice
  vinegar*
1 stalk celery, chopped

½ teaspoon dried basil
¼ teaspoon dried oregano

Combine all ingredients in a blender. Blend on high speed until
smooth. Store in the refrigerator, and use within a few days.

For 12 servings:

Per serving:
11 calories / 0.3 gm protein / † gm fat / † gm sat. fat /
0.0 mg cholesterol

---

* Seasoned rice vinegar can be bought at Oriental food stores.
† Less than 0.05 gm

Supper

OVEN FRIES

This is a recipe for oven French fries.
They taste great and are much better for
you than their deep-fried counterparts.

5–6 large potatoes
  1 tablespoon oil

1. Cut (unpeeled) potatoes lengthwise into ½-inch widths.
2. Spread potato wedges on a 12-by-16-inch pan.
3. Drizzle the oil over the potatoes. Use your hands to coat the potatoes thoroughly with oil.
4. In a 400-degree-F. oven, cook the potatoes under the broiler for 10 minutes.
5. Put the pan on the bottom shelf of the oven and bake for 20 minutes, or until potatoes are tender.

Note: To make a double batch, use 2 pans. Place 1 pan in the oven and 1 under the broiler. After 10 minutes, switch the pans. Ten minutes later, put the pan from the broiler into the oven and bake both pans for an additional 10 minutes.

For 4 servings:

Per serving:
225 calories / 4.1 gm protein / 3.6 gm fat / 0.5 gm sat. fat / 0.0 mg cholesterol

POTATO-CORN CHOWDER

This is a great soup for a cold evening.

2 teaspoons oil
½ cup chopped onion
7 cups finely diced potatoes
    (½-inch dice)
4 cups water
1 teaspoon granulated garlic

1 teaspoon oregano
1 teaspoon salt
4 cups corn kernels
¼ teaspoon black pepper
    (or to taste)
½ teaspoon salt (or to taste)

1. Heat the oil, and sauté the onion in it for 2 minutes.
2. Add potatoes, water, garlic, oregano, and salt. Bring to a boil and simmer for 12 minutes, or until potatoes are soft. Add corn.
3. Remove 2 cups of the soup from the pot and puree it in a blender or food processor. Return pureed soup to the pot. Add salt and pepper and heat well. Serve hot.

For seven servings:

Per serving:
204 calories / 5.3 gm protein / 1.5 gm fat / 0.2 gm sat. fat / 0.0 mg cholesterol

"REFRIED" BEANS

These beans, unlike traditional refried beans,
do not contain any oil. They are great served on flour
tortillas, with tomatoes, lettuce, and salsa.

4 cups cooked or canned
    pinto beans
1 teaspoon salt (or to taste)
1 tablespoon chili powder

½ teaspoon granulated garlic
1 cup chopped onion
¼ cup plus 1 tablespoon water

1. In a food processor, with a metal blade, blend beans with salt, chili powder, and garlic until smooth.
2. In a 2-quart saucepan, "sauté" the onion in ¼ cup of the water for 3 minutes. Add the additional tablespoon of water and "sauté" 1 minute more.
3. Add the beans and stir constantly over high heat until hot.

For 8 ½-cup servings:

Per serving:
129 calories / 7.5 gm protein / 0.6 gm fat / 0.1 gm sat. fat / 0.0 mg cholesterol

SUPER-SAUCY EGGPLANT LASAGNA

*This lasagna is great served with a
green salad and French bread.*

1 pound lasagna noodles,
    cooked and drained

Sauce:

1 tablespoon olive oil
1 cup chopped onion
½ cup chopped bell pepper
4 cups finely diced peeled
    eggplant
    juice from stewed tomatoes
    (if necessary to prevent
    sticking)
1 cup sliced mushrooms
6 cups stewed tomatoes

12 ounces tomato paste
2 teaspoons granulated garlic
2 teaspoons dried basil
1 teaspoon dried oregano
1 teaspoon salt (or to taste)
½ teaspoon dried thyme
¼ teaspoon black pepper
2 tablespoons brown sugar
2 tablespoons soy sauce
    (preferably shoyu)

Tofu filling:

1 10½-ounce package firm
    silken tofu
¼ teaspoon granulated garlic
¼ teaspoon salt

To prepare sauce:

1. In a heavy 4-quart saucepan, heat the olive oil and sauté the onion in it for 1 minute.
2. Add the bell pepper and sauté 1 minute more.
3. Add the eggplant, cover, and cook on medium heat for 5 minutes, stirring often. Add some of the juice from the tomatoes, if necessary, to prevent sticking.
4. Add the mushrooms and cook 1 minute, uncovered.
5. Stir in the remaining sauce ingredients. Cook over low heat until hot.

To prepare filling:

1. In a small bowl, use a fork to mash the tofu with the garlic and salt until it has the consistency of cottage cheese.

To assemble:

1. Put a layer of noodles in an oiled 12-by-16-inch pan (or a pan of equivalent area). Cover with a generous layer of sauce. Repeat, this time putting half of the tofu over the sauce. Repeat, putting the remaining tofu on top.
2. Bake lasagna in a 350-degree oven for 10–15 minutes, or until hot.

For 10 servings:

Per serving:
381 calories / 13.4 gm protein / 8.0 gm fat* / 1.3 gm sat. fat /
0.4 mg cholesterol

---

* Although moderately high in total fat per serving, the dish derives only 19 percent of its calories from fat and only 3 percent of calories from saturated fat.

VEGETABLE PIZZA

*This pizza is low in fat because the cheese has
been omitted, but it is still quite delicious
and is a hit at my house.*

Crust:

2 teaspoons sugar *or* honey
2 cups warm water
2 packages active dry yeast
2 teaspoons salt
2 teaspoons olive oil (plus ½
   for the rising bowl and 3
   teaspoons, 1 for each pan)

2 cups all-purpose or
   unbleached white flour
2¾–3½ cups whole-wheat flour
   cornmeal (for dusting pans)

Sauce:*

50 ounces tomato puree
1 tablespoon sugar
1–2 teaspoons oregano
1–2 teaspoons basil

1 teaspoon thyme
1 teaspoon granulated garlic
1 teaspoon salt
¼–½ teaspoon black pepper

Toppings (use any of the following that you desire):

sliced mushrooms
chopped bell peppers
chopped onion

grated summer squash
sliced tomatoes
olives (high in fat; use sparingly)

To prepare crust:

1. In a large bowl, dissolve the sugar in the water. Sprinkle in the
   yeast and let sit for 5 minutes, or until foamy.
2. Stir in the salt and oil.

---

* This pizza has a lot of sauce, which helps to replace the cheese. If you don't like so much
sauce on your pizza, save the rest for another meal.

3. Using a large spoon, stir in the white flour, and as much of the whole-wheat flour as you can to make a firm dough.
4. Turn out the dough onto a floured board, and knead for 8–10 minutes, or until the dough is smooth and elastic. Add additional whole-wheat flour to keep the dough from sticking to your hands.
5. Place the dough in a bowl that has been oiled with ½ teaspoon of olive oil, and cover with a damp cloth. Let the dough rise for 1½–2 hours, or until doubled in bulk.
6. Punch down the dough and cut it into 3 equal pieces. On a floured board, roll each piece into a 12-inch circle. Place the pieces of dough in 12-inch pizza pans that have been oiled (1 teaspoon of oil per pan) and lightly dusted with cornmeal.

To prepare sauce:

1. Combine all the sauce ingredients in a 2-quart saucepan, adding the spices to taste.
2. Heat the sauce over high heat until hot.

To assemble pizzas:

1. Spread the sauce evenly on the pizza crusts.
2. Place the toppings over the sauce.
3. Bake at 400 degrees F. for 15–20 minutes, or until the crust is lightly browned.

For 3 12-inch pizzas, or 12 large servings:

Per serving:
254 calories / 9.4 gm protein / 1.9 gm fat / 0.3 gm sat. fat / 0.0 mg cholesterol

VEGETARIAN CHILI

*Serve with a green salad and
fat-free crackers for a hearty meal.*

1 cup chopped onion
¼ cup water
⅓ cup finely chopped celery
⅔ cup finely chopped carrot
2 cups corn kernels
1 15-ounce can tomato sauce
1 6-ounce can tomato paste
1 4-ounce can mushrooms

5 cups cooked or canned
   pinto beans
1 cup cooking liquid from
   the beans
1 tablespoon molasses
3 tablespoons chili powder
   (or to taste)
1 teaspoon salt (or to taste)

1. "Sauté" the onion in water for 2 minutes.
2. Add the celery and carrot and "sauté" 2–3 minutes more, or until
   the vegetables are tender.
3. Stir in remaining ingredients and heat over high heat until hot.

For 6 servings:

Per serving:
317 calories / 16.1 gm protein / 2.3 gm fat / 0.4 gm sat. fat /
0.0 mg cholesterol

Desserts and Breads

APPLE CRISP

*This sweet dessert is similar to apple pie,
but much easier to make.*

Filling:

8 cups cored, peeled, and
sliced applies (tart, juicy
apples are best)
juice of ½ a lemon (⅛ cup)

2 tablespoons honey
1 tablespoon cornstarch
2 teaspoons cinnamon
1 teaspoon nutmeg

Topping:

1 cup whole-wheat flour
⅓ cup rolled oats
⅓ cup brown sugar
¼ cup chopped pecans
½ teaspoon cinnamon

½ teaspoon nutmeg
¼ teaspoon salt
1 tablespoon oil
2 tablespoons honey
juice of ½ a lemon

1. Preheat oven to 350 degrees F.
2. Combine the filling ingredients, and put the filling into a 9-inch pie pan (or a pan of equivalent area).
3. In a small bowl, combine the flour, oats, sugar, pecans, cinnamon, nutmeg, and salt.
4. Stir the oil, honey, and lemon juice into the flour mixture and blend well, using your hands.
5. Sprinkle the topping over the filling.
6. Bake for 30 minutes, or until the apples are soft and the topping is lightly browned.

For 8 servings:

Per serving:
252 calories / 3.2 gm protein / 5.3 gm fat / 0.7 gm sat. fat / 0.0 mg cholesterol

APPLESAUCE MUFFINS

*These sweet muffins are
delicious when they are fresh out of the oven,
and also good in sack lunches.*

Dry ingredients:

1½ cups whole-wheat flour
½ cup unbleached white
    flour
¼ cup wheat germ
1½ teaspoons baking soda
1½ teaspoons baking powder

1 teaspoon cinnamon
½ teaspoon nutmeg
¼ teaspoon allspice
¼ teaspoon ginger

Wet ingredients:

1 cup applesauce
⅔ cup honey
⅓ cup water

1 tablespoon oil
1 tablespoon vanilla

1. Preheat oven to 350 degrees F., and lightly oil a 12-muffin muffin pan.
2. In a medium-sized bowl, combine the dry ingredients.
3. In a separate bowl, beat together the wet ingredients.
4. Using a large spoon, fold together the wet and dry mixtures, being careful not to overmix.
5. Spoon the batter into the lightly oiled muffin pan.
6. Bake for 20 minutes, or until a wooden pick inserted in the center comes out clean.

For 12 servings:

Per serving (1 muffin):
170 calories / 3.0 gm protein / 1.7 gm fat / 0.3 gm sat. fat / 0.0 mg cholesterol

Variation:

PINEAPPLE UPSIDE-DOWN CAKE

 1 tablespoon margarine
¼ cup honey
 1 20-ounce can crushed
    pineapple

1. Lightly oil a 9-by-12-inch pan.
2. Melt margarine in a small pan with the honey. Pour the honey-margarine mixture into the prepared 9-by-12-inch pan.
3. Drain the pineapple and spoon it over the honey mixture. (Save the juice to use in the batter.)
4. Prepare batter for Applesauce Muffins, omitting the wheat germ and allspice, and using the pineapple juice in place of water.
5. Spoon the batter into the pan and carefully spread it out so that it is even.
6. Bake in a 350-degree-F. oven for 30 minutes, or until a wooden pick inserted in the middle comes out clean.
7. Cool in the pan for at least 30 minutes, and then invert the cake onto a serving platter.

For 12 large servings:

Per serving:
220 calories / 2.5 gm protein / 2.4 gm fat / 0.5 gm sat. fat / 0.0 mg cholesterol

BANANA-OAT MUFFINS

These are my favorite muffins.

Dry ingredients:

1½ cups whole-wheat flour
1 cup unbleached white flour
1 teaspoon nutmeg
¼ cup chopped walnuts
2 teaspoons baking soda

Wet ingredients:

1½ cup honey or Fruitsource*
1 cup mashed banana
2 teaspoons oil
1 teaspoon vanilla
½ cup water

Topping:

1 teaspoon cinnamon
¾ cup rolled oats
½ cup brown sugar
1 tablespoon oil

1. Mix together dry ingredients.
2. Beat together wet ingredients.
3. Stir together topping ingredients.
4. Mix together wet and dry mixtures and spoon into a lightly oiled 12-muffin muffin pan.
5. Sprinkle batter with topping.
6. Bake in a 375-degree-F. oven until the top springs back when lightly touched (about 25 minutes).

For 12 servings:

Per serving (1 muffin):
238 calories / 4.6 gm protein / 4.3 gm fat / 0.6 gm sat. fat / 0.0 mg cholesterol

---

* Fruitsource is a sweetener that is made out of grape-juice concentrate and rice syrup. It can be found at natural-food stores and used in place of honey.

CHOCOLATE-BROWNIE CAKE

This dessert is a cross between brownies and cake.
It is rich, but much lower in fat than most cakes.

1 cup whole-wheat flour
⅓ cup unbleached white
   flour
½ cup cocoa *or* carob
   powder* (or ¼ cup of
   each)
2½ teaspoons baking powder
1¼ cups water
¾ cup brown sugar
½ cup applesauce

¼ cup honey
2 teaspoons vanilla
¼ teaspoon rum, orange, *or*
   lemon extract (optional)
2 tablespoons dark
   (semisweet) chocolate
   chips†
2 tablespoons slivered
   almonds *or* chopped
   walnuts

1. Sift together the cocoa and baking powder (to remove lumps), and then stir into the flours, using a wire whisk.
2. Dissolve the brown sugar in the water, and beat in the applesauce, honey, vanilla, and flavoring (if used).
3. Pour wet ingredients into the flour mixture and whisk thoroughly.
4. Pour batter into a lightly oiled 9-inch-square pan (or a 9-inch round pan) and sprinkle with chocolate chips and nuts.
5. Bake in a 325-degree-F. oven for 35–40 minutes, or until a wooden pick inserted near the center comes out clean.

For 16 servings:

Per serving:
115 calories / 2.1 gm protein / 1.4 gm fat / 0.5 gm sat. fat /
0.0 mg cholesterol

---

* Carob powder is a nonfat substitute for cocoa powder. Because it is naturally sweet, it makes a sweeter dessert than chocolate. It contains no fat, caffeine, or added sugar. A good alternative for people who are allergic to chocolate, it can be found at natural-food stores.
† If you are avoiding dairy products, look for dark (semisweet) chocolate chips that contain no milk.

CHOCOLATE-CHIP CRANBERRY COOKIES

*Chocolate-chip cookies usually have large amounts
of butter, nuts, and chocolate chips, which are all
very high in fat. In these cookies, I have greatly
reduced the amount of fatty ingredients, and I have
added cranberries, which provide a unique flavor.*

2 cups whole-wheat flour
1 cup unbleached white flour
½ cup brown sugar
⅓ cup chocolate chips
2 tablespoons walnuts
1 teaspoon baking powder
½ teaspoon baking soda
¼ teaspoon salt

1½ cups whole cranberries (½ of a 12-ounce package)
½ cup honey
½ cup grape juice *or* any other fruit juice
3 tablespoons applesauce
1 tablespoon oil

1. In a bowl, combine the flours, sugar, chocolate chips, walnuts, baking powder, baking soda, and salt. Gently stir in the cranberries.
2. In a separate bowl, beat together the honey, juice, applesauce, and oil.
3. Preheat the oven to 325 degrees F.
4. Pour the honey mixture over the flour mixture, and stir together until the dry ingredients are moistened (don't overmix, or the dough will become tough).
5. Using 2 tablespoons, spoon cookie dough onto cookie sheets that have been sprayed with cooking spray or lightly oiled.
6. Bake the cookies for 15 minutes, or until the bottoms are light brown and the tops spring back when lightly touched.

For 24 servings, 1 medium-sized cookie each:

Per serving (1 cookie):
119 calories / 2.2 gm protein / 1.9 gm fat / 0.6 gm sat. fat / 0.0 mg cholesterol

CORN BREAD

*I love corn bread, but I don't like the large amounts
of eggs and milk in most corn breads. So I did some
experimenting and here's what I came up with. It's sweet, and
much more substantial than corn bread made from a mix.*

1 cup cornmeal (stone-ground is best)
1 cup Masa Harina* *or* an additional cup of cornmeal
½ cup whole-wheat flour
1 teaspoon baking soda
1 teaspoon baking powder
¾ teaspoon salt
⅓ cup molasses
2 cups water
1 teaspoon oil (for oiling the pan)

1. Preheat the oven to 400 degrees F.
2. Whisk together the cornmeal, Masa Harina, flour, baking soda, baking powder, and salt.
3. Beat together molasses and water.
4. Whisk together wet and dry mixtures, and pour into an oiled 9-inch-square pan.
5. Bake for 25 minutes, or until the top is lightly browned.

For 16 servings:

Per serving:
97 calories / 2.0 gm protein / 0.7 gm fat / 0.1 gm sat. fat /
0.0 mg cholesterol

* Masa Harina, a flour made from corn hominy, can be found at most grocery stores.

GINGERBREAD COOKIES

*Kids love to help cut out these cookies, and
they enjoy eating them even more than they would
otherwise because they helped make them.*

2 cups whole-wheat flour
1½ cups unbleached white
    flour
1 teaspoon baking soda
1 teaspoon ginger
½ teaspoon cinnamon
¼ teaspoon cloves *or*
    allspice

¼ teaspoon salt
½ cup molasses
½ cup brown sugar
2 tablespoons canola oil
2 tablespoons applesauce
7 tablespoons water

Icing:
¼ cup powdered sugar, sifted
¼ teaspoon lemon extract
    (optional)
1–3 teaspoons water

1. Mix together the flours, baking soda, ginger, cinnamon, cloves, and salt.
2. With a fork, beat together the molasses, brown sugar, oil, and applesauce; then beat in the water.
3. Combine the molasses and flour mixtures. Blend them together well, using a spoon and, if necessary, your hands.
4. Preheat the oven to 350 degrees F.
5. On a floured board, roll out the dough ¼ inch thick and cut with cookie cutters.
6. Place the cookies on cookie sheets that have been sprayed with cooking spray or lightly oiled. Bake the cookies for 8 minutes, or until the dough springs back when lightly touched. Let cool on a wire rack.
7. Using a fork, stir together the powdered sugar, flavoring, and enough water to make a thin icing.

8. Drizzle the icing over the cookies. Let the icing dry, and then store the cookies in an airtight container.

For 48 servings, 1 2-to-3-inch cookie each:

Per serving (1 cookie):
58 calories / 1.1 gm protein / 0.7 gm fat / 0.1 gm sat. fat / 0.0 mg cholesterol

---

"MUD" COOKIES

These are dark, moist chocolate cookies.

1 cup whole-wheat flour
⅓ cup unbleached white flour
½ cup cocoa *or* carob powder
   (or ¼ cup of each)
¾ cup brown sugar
1 teaspoon baking soda

1 teaspoon baking powder
⅓ cup raisins (optional)
⅔ cup applesauce
1⅓ cup fruit juice, such as
   grape, orange, or apple
1 tablespoon canola oil

1. Preheat the oven to 325 degrees F.
2. In a medium-sized bowl, mix together the flours, cocoa powder, brown sugar, baking soda, baking powder, and raisins (if used).
3. In a separate bowl, mix together the applesauce, fruit juice, and oil.
4. Using a wire whisk, vigorously mix the wet and dry ingredients to produce a very moist batter.
5. Using a tablespoon, drop the batter onto lightly oiled cookie sheets.
6. Bake for 15–20 minutes, or until the tops of the cookies bounce back when lightly touched.

For 36 servings, 1 cookie each:

Per serving (1 cookie):
51 calories / 0.9 gm protein / 0.6 gm fat / 0.2 gm sat. fat /
0.0 mg cholesterol

Notes

Introduction

Page

xxii established during youth: Lloyd Kolbe, "An Essential Strategy to Improve the Health and Education of Americans," *Preventive Medicine*, vol. 22 (1993), pp. 544–60.

xxii born healthy: Walter M. Bortz II, M.D., *We Live Too Short and Die Too Long* (New York: Bantam Books, 1991), p. 76. Dr. Knowles quoted by the author.

xxii 10 leading causes of death: National Center for Health Statistics, Centers for Disease Control and Prevention (Hyattsville, Md.), "Latest Rankings of Causes of Death," 1991, unpublished.

xxiii up to 70 percent: E. Woteki and P. Thomas, eds., *Eat for Life* (Washington, D.C.: National Academy Press, 1992), p. 68.

xxiii *what they ate during their childhood:* Neal Barnard, M.D., *Food for Life* (New York: Harmony Books, 1993), p. 71.

xxiii develop . . . cancer as adults: P. Mills, W. L. Beeson, R. L. Phillips, and G. E. Fraser, "Cohort Study Diet, Lifestyle, and Prostate Cancer in Adventist Men," *Cancer*, vol. 64 (1989), pp. 598–604.

xxiv lifetime eating habits: Christine Williams and Ernst Wynder, "A Child Health Report Card: 1992," *Preventive Medicine*, vol. 22 (1993), pp. 604–28.

xxiv *prostate cancer:* R. L. Phillips, "Role of Lifestyle and Dietary Habits in Risk of Cancer Among Seventh-Day Adventists," *Cancer Research*, vol. 35 (1975), pp. 3513–22.

xxiv *raised as vegetarians:* E. Woteki and P. Thomas, eds., *Eat for Life* (Washington, D.C.: National Academy Press, 1992), p. 71.

xxiv *second generation:* John H. Weisburger, Ph.D., "Mechanism of Action of Diet as a Carcinogen," presented at the American Cancer Society and National Cancer Institute National Conference on Nutrition in Cancer, June 29–July 1, 1978, Seattle, Washington, published in *Cancer*, May supple. 1979.

xxiv *their daughters:* T. Hirayama, "Epidemiology of Breast Cancer with Special reference to the Role of Diet," *Preventive Medicine*, vol. 7 (1978), pp. 173–95.

xxiv Scottish women: Dr. Peter Boyle, Director, Division of Epidemiology and Biostatistics, Instituto Europeo di Oncologia, Sr I, via Ripananti 332/10, 20140, Milan, Italy.

xxiv "unknown" protective factor: P. Boyle and C. Robertson, "Breast Cancer and Colon Cancer Incidence in Females in Scotland, 1960–84," *Journal of the National Cancer Institute*, vol. 79, no. 6 (Dec. 1987), pp. 1175–79. Dr. Boyle later concluded that the protective factor was their childhood diet. Unpublished communication from Clara L. Horn at the American Health Foundation, 1994.

xxiv later . . . menstruation: personal communication from Dr. Hans Diehl, Lifestyle Medicine Institute, Loma Linda, Calif.

xxv Another explanation: personal communication from John H. Weisburger, Ph.D., American Health Foundation, Valhalla, N.Y.

xxv A Harvard study: W. Willett et al.: "Dietary Fat and the Risk of Breast Cancer," *New England Journal of Medicine*, vol. 316 (1987), pp. 22–28.

xxv *These Italian women:* P. Toniolo, "Calorie-providing Nutrients and Risk of Breast Cancer, *Journal of the National Cancer Institute*, vol. 81 (1989), pp. 278–86.

xxvi almost none of AHA's grant money: AHA President Suzanne Oparil, M.D., speech at Bogalusa Heart Study conference, April 28, 1994, New Orleans, La.

xxvi misplaced emphasis: C. B. Esselstyn, Jr., "Beyond Surgery," *Surgery*, vol. 110 (1991), pp. 923–27 Also personal communication from C. B. Esselstyn, Jr.

xxvi ". . . edge of a cliff . . .": D. Burkitt, "An Approach to the Reduction of the Most Common Western Cancers," *Archives of Surgery*, vol. 126 (1991), pp. 345–47.

xxx *not* essential nutrients: G. Berenson, Editorial: "Cholesterol, Myth vs Reality in Pediatric Practice," *American Journal of Diseases of Children*, vol. 147 (April 1993), pp. 371–73.

xxx "diseases of nutritional extravagance": personal communication from T. Colin Campbell, Ph.D., Cornell University.

xxxiii in most teenagers: *Arteriosclerosis and Thrombosis*, vol. 13 (1993), pp. 1291–98.

Chapter 1
Myth One: Controlling Cholesterol Can Wait

4 (42 percent of calories): "Coronary Artery Disease Prevention: Cholesterol, a Pediatric Perspective," an American Health Foundation Monograph, *Preventive Medicine* (New York: Academic Press, 1989), p. 357.

5 *only one* major risk factor: W. C. Roberts, "Atherosclerotic Risk Factors—Are There Ten or Is There Only One?" *American Journal of Cardiology*, vol. 64 (1989), pp. 552–54.

6 ". . . heart attack in Framingham . . .": personal communication from Dr. William Castelli.

6 ". . . consumed by three-quarters of the people": Neal Barnard, *The Power of Your Plate* (Summertown, Tenn.: Book Publishing Co., 1990), p. 16.

7 ". . . Of the 5.3 billion . . .": William Castelli, M.D., interview by *McCall's Good Health* suppl. Fall/Winter 1993, p. 52.

7 seven years longer: personal communication from Dr. Hans Diehl, Lifestyle Medicine Institute, Loma Linda, Calif.

12 Korean: W. Enos et al., "Coronary Disease Among United States Soldiers Killed in Action in Korea," *Journal of the American Medical Association*, vol. 152 (1953), pp. 1090–93.

12 Vietnam: J. McNamara et al. "Coronary Artery Disease in Combat Casualties in Vietnam." *Journal of the American Medical Association*, vol. 216 (1971), pp. 1185–87.

12 "We have come to recognize . . .": Committee on Nutrition, *Pediatric Nutrition Handbook* (Elk Grove Village, Ill.: American Academy of Pediatrics, 1992), p. v.

13 cholesterol levels of the elderly: D. Leaf, "Lipid Disorders: Applying New Guidelines to Your Older Patients," *Geriatrics*, vol. 49 (1994), pp. 35–41.

13 second-birthday: C. Attwood, "Cholesterol Screening: How Much Is Enough?," *Pediatric Management*, Nov. 1991, pp. 25–29.

15 St. Paul's School: C. H. Ford, "An Institutional Approach to the Dietary Regulation of Blood Cholesterol in Adolescent Males," *Preventive Medicine*, vol. 1 (1972), pp. 426–45.

17 Hydrogenated fat is made: "Nutrition Advisor," *Physician and Sportsmedicine*, vol. 22, no. 3 (March 1994), p. 36.

18 30,000 heart disease deaths: W. Willett. "Trans Fatty Acids: Are the Effects Only Marginal?," *American Journal of Public Health*, vol. 84, no. 5 (May 1994), pp. 722–24.

Chapter 2
Myth Two: Controlling Obesity Can Wait

21 "Obesity . . . is of growing concern . . .": Ernst L. Wynder, M.D., "A Child Health Report Card: 1992," presented at conference: The Health Status of American Children and Youth, Oct. 5, 1993, American Health Foundation, New York.

21 "Health is three things . . .": Walter M. Bortz II, M.D., *We Live Too Short and Die Too Long* (New York: Bantam Books, 1991), p. 81.

22 each additional hour: C. Conti, *Heart Disease and High Cholesterol* (Reading, Mass.: Addison-Wesley, 1992), p. 77.

22 23 hours weekly: Lawrence Kutner, "How Much Television Is TOO Much for Your Kids?" *New York Times*, July 4, 1993.

22 5 hours of TV per day: personal communication from Dr. Frederick Kaye, Tallahassee, Fl.

22 41 percent: Jerry Bishop, "TV Advertising Aimed at Kids Is Filled with Fat," *Wall Street Journal*, Nov. 9, 1993, p. B1.

23 chubby infants . . . obese adults: E. Charney et al., "Childhood Antecedents of Adult Obesity. Do Chubby Infants Become Obese Adults?" *New England Journal of Medicine*, vol. 295, no. 1 (July 1, 1976), pp. 6–9.

23 his classic book: Dr. Benjamin Spock, *Dr. Spock's Baby and Child Care* (New York: Pocket Books, 1992).

24 consultant to sports associations: personal communication from Bruce Woolley, Pharm.D., Department of Food Science and Nutrition, Brigham Young University, Provo, Utah.

25 adolescent obesity in males: A. Must et al., "Long-term Morbidity and Mortality of Overweight Adolescents: A Follow-up of the Harvard Growth Study of 1922–1935," *New England Journal of Medicine*, vol. 327 (1992), pp. 1350–55.

25 excessive numbers of fat cells: W. Clarke and R. Lauer, "Does Childhood Obesity Track into Adulthood?," *Critical Reviews in Food Science and Nutrition*, vol. 33, nos. 4/5 (1993), pp. 423–30.

26 more obese American children: C. L. Shear et al., "Secular Trends in Obesity in Early Life: The Bogalusa Heart Study," *American Journal of Pediatric Health*, vol. 78 (1988), pp. 75–77. Gortmaker et al., "Increasing Pediatric Obesity," *American Journal of Diseases of Children*, vol. 141 (1987), p. 535.

26 ages of 25 and 30: Paul Raeburn, Associated Press, March 18, 1994. R. J. Kuczmarski, Dr. P.H., R.D., "Increasing Prevalence of Overweight Among U.S. Adults," *JAMA*, vol. 272 (1994), pp. 205–11.

27 a 1991 study: T. L. Burns et al., "Increased Familial Cardiovascular Mortality in Obese Schoolchildren: The Muscatine Ponderosity Family Study," *Pediatrics*, vol. 89, no. 2 (February 1992), pp. 262–68.

29 "the kids won't change": Neal Barnard, *The Power of Your Plate* (Summertown, Tenn.: Book Publishing Co., 1990), p. 92. Dr. William Connor interviewed by author.

29 modern malady: S. Boyd Eaton, M.D., Marjorie Shostak, and Melvin Konner, M.D., Ph.D., *The Paleolithic Prescription: A Program of Diet & Exercise and a Design for Living* (New York: Harper & Row, 1988), p. 45.

31 "flywheel effect": personal communication from Terry Shintani, University of Hawaii.

34 8 out of 10: T. Romieu, "Energy Intake and Other Determinants of Relative Weight, *American Journal of Clinical Nutrition*, vol. 47 (1988), pp. 406–12.

Chapter 3
Myth Three: The "Fat Taste" Is Natural and Inborn

37 "If you let . . .": L. L. Birch, "Children's Preferences for High-Fat Foods," *Nutritional Review*, vol. 50, no. 9 (Sept. 1992), pp. 249–55.

38 offering ice cream: Dr. Benjamin Spock, *Dr. Spock's Baby and Child Care* (New York: Pocket Books, 1992), p. 357.

38 ". . . patients of tomorrow": Neal Barnard, M.D., *Food for Life* (New York: Harmony Books, 1993), p. 160.

39 8 to 12 weeks: R. D. Mattes, "Fat Preference and Adherence to a Reduced-Fat Diet," *American Journal of Clinical Nutrition*, vol. 57, no. 3 (March 1993), pp. 373–81.

40 galanin . . . encourages fat consumption: Sarah Leibowitz, "Central Physiological Determinants of Eating Behavior and Body Weight," unpublished, 1994.

40 causes animals to eat *less*: L. Lin, D. Gehlert, D. York, and G. Bray, "Effect of Enterostatin on the Feeding Responses to Galanin and NPY," *Obesity Research*, vol. 1, no. 3 (May 1993), pp. 186–92.

Chapter 4
Myth Four: Small Reductions in Fat Will Do

43 appease the public: Peter Radetsky, "The Live-Longer Diet," *Longevity*, May 1994.

44 reduced to 10–15 percent: D. Ornish et al., "Can Lifestyle Changes Reverse Coronary Heart Disease?," *Lancet*, vol. 336 (1990), pp. 129–33.

44 6 studies: Dean Ornish, M.D., letter to the editor, *JAMA*, vol. 267, no. 3 (January 15, 1992), p. 362; B. G. Brown et al., "Regression of Coronary Artery Disease as a Result of Intensive Lipid-lowering Therapy in Men with High Levels of Apolipoprotein B," *New England Journal of Medicine*, vol. 323 (1990), pp. 1289–98; H. Buchwald et al., "Effect of Partial Ileal Bypass Surgery on Mortality and Morbidity from Coronary Heart Disease on Patients with Hypercholesterolemia," *New England Journal of Medicine*, vol. 323 (1990), pp. 946–55; L. Cashin-Hemphill et al., "Beneficial Effects of Colestipol-Niacin on Coronary Atherosclerosis: A 4-Year Follow-up," *JAMA*, vol. 264 (1990), pp. 3013–17; J. P. Kane et al., "Regression of Coronary Atherosclerosis During Treatment of Familial Hypercholesterolemia with Combined Drug Regimens, *JAMA*, vol. 264 (1990), pp. 3007–12; R. I. Levy et al., "The Influence of Changes in Lipid Values Induced by Cholestyramine and Diet on Progression of Coronary Artery Disease: Results of NHLBI Type II Coronary Intervention Study," *Circulation*, vol. 69 (1984), pp. 325–37.

45 ". . . scare people off": personal communication from Bonnie Liebman, Center for Science in the Public Interest, Washington, D.C., 1994.

45 admitted privately: Adult and Child Treatment Panels, personal communication from National Cholesterol Education Program, 1989.

46 "Your panel could . . .": personal communication from the Center for Science in the Public Interest, Washington, D.C., February 8, 1994.

46 "You can't handle the truth!": Aaron Sorkin, *A Few Good Men*, playscript (New York: Samuel French, 1990), p. 116.

46 A 1992 study: N. Barnard and D. Ornish, "Adherence and Acceptability of a Low-Fat, Vegetarian Diet Among Cardiac Patients," *Journal of Cardiopulmonary Rehabilitation*, vol. 12, no. 6 (Nov.–Dec. 1992), pp. 423–31.

47 "The scientific evidence . . .": quoted in C. Woteki and P. Thomas, eds., *Eat for Life* (Washington, D.C.: National Academy Press, 1992), p. 22.

48 500,000 Americans die: *The Nation's No. 1 Health Problem*, Robert Wood Johnson Foundation, Communications Department, P.O. Box 2316, Princeton, N.J. 08543-2316.

48 $238 billion: Associated Press, "Substance Abuse Kills 500,000 a Year, Study Says," *Rocky Mountain News*, October 22, 1993.

Chapter 5
Myth Five: Children's Diets Are Getting Better

50 a sad face: *Time*, March 26, 1984, cover.

52 42 percent of its calories: "Coronary Artery Disease Prevention: Cholesterol, a Pediatric Perspective," *Preventive Medicine* (New York: Academic Press, 1989), p. 357.

52 "They are tired . . .": Richard Gibson, "Back to Fat," *Wall Street Journal*, April 15, 1993.

52 "Fat is needed . . ." Richard Woodbury, "The Great Fast-Food Pig-out," *Time*, June 28, 1993.

53 Back at the White House: "Veggie Bits," *Vegetarian Journal*, vol. 13, no. 5 (Sept.–Oct. 1994), p. 22.

Chapter 6
Myth Six: Meat Is Needed for Protein and Iron

56 obtain two-thirds: Frances Moore Lappe, *Diet for a Small Planet* (New York: Ballantine Books, 1982), pp. 121–22.

56 only 10.8 precent: J. Chen, C. L. Campbell, J. Li, and R. Peto, *Diet, Life-Style and Mortality in China: A Study of the Characteristics of 65 Chinese Counties* (Ithaca, N.Y.: Cornell University Press, 1990), p. 62.

56 replaced with soybean protein: C. R. Sirtori, E. Agradi, F. Conti, O. Mantero, and E. Gatti, "Soybean-Protein Diet in the Treatment of Type-II Hyperlipoproteinemia," *Lancet*, vol. 5, no. 1 (Feb. 1977), pp. 275–77.

56 After 8 weeks: G. C. Descavish, C. Ceredi, A. Gaddi, M. C. Benassi et al., "Multicentre Study of Soybean Protein Diet for Outpatient Hypercholesterolemic Patients," *Lancet*, vol. 4, no. 2 (Oct. 1980), pp. 709–12.

56 higher rates of heart disease: "The Problem With Protein," *Nutrition Action Healthletter* (Center for Science in the Public Interest, Washington, D.C.), June 1993.

57 ". . . risk of cancers . . .": National Academy of Sciences, *Diet, Nutrition, and Cancer* (Washington, D.C.: National Academy Press, 1982), p. 102.

57 88,751 women: Jeremy Rifkin, *Beyond Beef* (New York: Dutton, 1992), p. 172.

57 ". . . should be zero": Gina Kolata, "Animal Fat Is Tied to Colon Cancer," *New York Times*, December 13, 1990.

57 simply changed from beef: Judith Mandelbaum-Schmidt, "The Chicken Breast Myth," *Health*, September, 1993.

57 study in Finland: J. T. Salonen, K. Nyyssonen, H. Korpela, J. Tuomilehto et al., "High Stored Iron Levels Are Associated with Excess Risk of Myocardial Infarction in Eastern Finnish Men," *Circulation*, vol. 86, no. 3 (Sept. 1992), pp. 803–11.

59 eat *only* 6–8 potatoes: Reed Mangels, Ph.D., R.D., "Potatoes as a Source of Protein," *Vegetarian Journal*, Jan.–Feb. 1994, p. 2.

61 ". . . eating themselves to death": Jeremy Rifkin, *Beyond Beef* (New York: Dutton, 1992), p. 174.

Chapter 7
Myth Seven: Milk Is Needed for Calcium and Protein

62 milk is not a desirable part: personal communication from Frank Oski, chairman, Department of Pediatrics, Johns Hopkins University School of Medicine, June 1994.

63 study by . . . Dosch: J. Karjalainen, J. M. Martin, M. Knip et al., "A Bovine

Albumin Peptide as a Possible Trigger of Insulin-Dependent Diabetes Mellitus," *New England Journal of Medicine*, vol. 327 (1992), pp. 302–7.

63 more diabetes is found: F. W. Scott, "Cow Milk and Insulin-dependent Diabetes: Is There a Relationship?," *American Journal of Clinical Nutrition*, vol. 51 (1990), pp. 489–91.

65 countries with the highest rates: "The Problem with Protein," *Nutrition Action Healthletter*, June 1993, p. 7.

66 Bantu women: A. Walker, "Osteoporosis and Calcium Deficiency," *American Journal of Clinical Nutrition*, vol. 16 (1965), p. 327.

66 nursing . . . 10 children: A. Walker, "The Influence of Numerous Pregnancies and Lactations on Bone Dimensions in South African Bantu and Caucasian Mothers," *Clinical Science*, vol. 42 (1972), p. 189.

66 Eskimos consume . . . high-protein diet: R. Mazess and W. Mather, "Bone Mineral Content of North Alaskan Eskimos," *American Journal of Clinical Nutrition*, vol. 27 (1974), pp. 916–25.

66 calcium . . . bone density: G. Kolata, "How Important Is Dietary Calcium in Preventing Osteoporosis?," *Science*, vol. 233 (1986), pp. 519–20.

66 non-dairy sources of calcium: Dr. Neal Barnard, *New York Times*, letter to the editor, September 11, 1993.

67 greens such as kale: Scott, "Cow Milk," pp. 489–91.

Chapter 8
Myth Eight: Low-Fat Diets Lack Vitamins and Minerals

70 "not yet been fully studied": A Natow and Jo-Ann Heslin, *The Antioxidant Counter* (New York: Pocket Books, 1994), p. xxvi.

70 "vitamin factories": Victoria Moran, *Compassion: the Ultimate Ethic* (Malaga, N.J.: American Vegan Society, 1991), p. 65.

71 provides *more* minerals and vitamins: J. T. Dwyer, "Nutritional Consequences of Vegetarianism," *Annual Review of Nutrition*, vol. 11 (1991), pp. 61–91.

71 daily needs of vitamin A: based on estimates from National Academy of Science, *Recommended Daily Allowances* (Washington, D.C.: National Academy Press, 10th ed., 1989).

72 5 servings: Julia Martin, "Good News! You *Can* Prevent a Heart Attack," *Family Circle*, Feb. 22, 1994, p. 64.

73 Pyramid: U.S. Department of Agriculture, U.S. Department of Health and Human Services, *The Food Guide Pyramid: A Guide to Daily Food Choices*. Consumer Information Center (Pueblo, Colo. 81009).

73 vitamins . . . may not be effective: "The Effect of Vitamin E and Beta Carotene on the Incidence of Lung Cancer and Other Cancers in Male Smokers," *New England Journal of Medicine*, vol. 330, no. 15 (April 14, 1994), p. 1029–35.

73 29,000 Finnish men: Gina Kolata, "Vitamin Supplements Are Seen as No Guard Against Diseases," *New York Times*, April 14, 1994.

73 premalignant colon polyps: Jerry E. Bishop, "Vitamins C, E and Beta Carotene Fail to Cut Risk of New Colon Polyps in Test," *Wall Street Journal*, July 21, 1994, p. B6.

73 *phytochemicals: Cancer Research*, vol. 52, suppl. (1992), p. 2085s.

75 B12-fortified soy milk: J. Dwyer, "Health Aspects of Vegetarian Diets," *American Journal of Clinical Nutrition*, vol. 48 (1988), pp. 712–38.

Chapter 9
Myth Nine: A Low-Fat Diet Means Limited Choices

78 stroll through a farmers' market: Victoria Moran, *Get the Fat Out*, Foreword by Suzanne Havala. (New York: Crown, 1994), pp. xvii–xviii.

78 ". . . small choice . . .": G. B. Harrison, *William Shakespeare: The Taming of the Shrew* (New York: Harcourt, Brace, and World, 1968), pp. 328–64.

79 10 . . . menus: personal communication from William Castelli, M.D.

79 grown in many varieties: Sheldon Margen, M.D., *The Wellness Encyclopedia of Food and Nutrition* (New York: Rebus, 1992), pp. 162–71.

80 20 distinctly different varieties: ibid., pp. 289–92.

81 bite-sized kiwi: Kerry Hannon, "New Fruits and Veggies for the '90s Cook," *U.S. News & World Report*, May 10, 1993, pp. 72–73.

Chapter 10
Myth Ten: Low-Fat Diets Retard Growth

83 included malnourished children: R. Kaplan and M. Toshima, "Does a Reduced Fat Diet Cause Retardation in Child Growth?," *Preventive Medicine*, vol. 21 (1952), pp. 33–52.

84 seriously flawed: ibid.

84 *greater* height: J. Sabate, K. D. Kindsted, R. Harris, and A. Sanchez, "Attained Height of Lacto-ovovegetarian Children and Adolescents." *European Journal of Clinical Nutrition*, vol. 45, no. 1 (1990), pp. 51–58.

84 did not affect ultimate height: J. Sabate, C. Llorca, and A. Sanchez, "Lower Height of Lacto-ovovegetarian Girls at Preadolescence: An Indicator of Physical Maturation Delay," *Journal of the American Diet Association*, vol. 92 (1992), pp. 1263–64.

84 same growth rate: Peter O. Kwiterovich, Jr., M.D., *The Johns Hopkins Complete Guide for Preventing and Reversing Heart Disease* (Rocklin, Calif.: Prima Publishing, 1993), p. 97.

85 Farm Study: J. O'Connell, M. Dibley, J. Sierra, B. Wallace, J. Marks, and R. Yip, "Growth of Vegetarian Children: The Farm Study," *Pediatrics*, vol. 84, no. 3 (Sept. 1989), pp. 475–81.

85 meat-based diet: M. G. Harding, and F. J. Stare, "Nutritional Studies of Vegetarians, I, Nutritional, Physical and Laboratory Studies," *American Journal of Clinical Nutrition*, vol. 2 (1954), p. 73.

86 no signs of growth retardation: V. D. Register and L. M. Sonnenberg, "The Vegetarian Diet," *Journal of the American Diet Association*, vol. 62 (1973), p. 253.

86 Israeli boys and girls: Kwiterovich, *Johns Hopkins Guide*, p. 97.

86 more proof: ibid., p. 97.

87 ". . . brain needs cholesterol . . .": ibid., p. 98.

88 full adult height is attained: personal communication from T. Colin Campbell, 1993.

Chapter 11
Myth Eleven: It's Obvious Which Foods Are High in Fat

89 foods served in the White House: Marian Burros, "Eating Well," *New York Times,* July 21, 1993, p. B1.

90 different concept: Connie Cass, "Gallic Fare Fades at White House," quoted Mr. Chambrin's statement to *USA Today,* Associated Press, March 5, 1994.

90 staff were fired: Marian Burros, "Eating Well" *New York Times,* Feb. 5, 1994.

90 replaced by . . . Scheib: Molly O'Neill, " 'Light Menu' for White House as a New Chef Takes Charge," *New York Times,* April 5, 1994.

90 Domino's Pizza: Harper's Index, *Harper's,* April 1994, p. 17.

91 from 3 to 4 per week: Kathleen Deveny, "Marketscan," *Wall Street Journal,* Oct. 14, 1993.

91 whole-egg products: *University of California at Berkeley Wellness Letter,* Aug. 1992.

91 essentially nonfat foods: Sheldon Margen, M.D., *The Wellness Encyclopedia of Food and Nutrition* (New York: Rebus, 1992), p. 460.

92 Low-fat vegetable sauces: Karol V. Menzie, "Vegetable Sauces Light Up an Entree," *Baltimore Sun,* March 30, 1994.

93 substitute for sour cream: C. Richard Conti, M.D., and Diana Tonnessen, *Heart Disease and High Cholesterol* (New York: Addison-Wesley, 1992), p. 43.

94 theater popcorn: Jane Hurley "Popcorn: Oil in a Day's Work," *Nutrition Action Healthletter,* April 1994, pp. 9–10.

Chapter 12
Myth Twelve: No One Knows What's *Really* Best for My Child

96 first large clinical studies: Multiple Risk Factor Intervention Trial Research Group, "Risk Factor Changes and Mortality Results," *JAMA,* vol. 248 (Sept. 1982), pp. 1465–77.

96 lowering cholesterol levels with drugs: M. H. Frick, O. Elo, K. Haapa et al., "Helsinki Heart Study: Primary-Prevention Trial with Gemfribrozil in Middle-aged Men with Dyslipidemia; Safety of Treatment, Changes in Risk Factors, and Incidence of Coronary Heart Disease," *New England Journal of Medicine,* vol. 317 (1987), pp. 1237–45.

97 doesn't prevent heart disease: T. J. Moore, "The Cholesterol Myth," *Atlantic,* Sept. 1989, pp. 37–70.

97 radio debate: personal communication from William Castelli, M.D.

97 absolute proof was found: P. Zeek, "Juvenile Arteriosclerosis," *Archives of Pathology,* vol. 10, pp. 417–46.

97 those consuming high-fat diets: Paula Einhorn, M.D., and Basil Rifkind, M.D., editorial, *American Journal of Diseases of Children,* vol. 147 (1993), pp. 373–75.

97 coronary-artery lesions: D. S. Freedman, W. P. Newman III, R. E. Tracy et al.,

"Black-White Differences in Aortic Fatty Streaks in Adolescence and Early Adulthood: The Bogalusa Heart Study," *Circulation*, vol. 77 (1988), pp. 856–64.

97 found at autopsies: W. P. Newman III, W. Wattigney, and G. S. Berenson, "Autopsy Studies in US Children and Adolescents: Relationship of Risk Factors to Atherosclerotic Lesions," *Annals of the New York Academy of Science*, vol. 623 (1991), pp. 16–25.

Chapter 13
4 Stages to an Ideal Diet

102 in stages: Neal Barnard, M.D., *Food for Life* (New York: Harmony Books, 1993), p. xviii.

102 each lasting several weeks: personal communication from T. Colin Campbell, Ph.D.

103 is not enough: J. Chen, C. L. Campbell, J. Li, and R. Peto, *Diet, Life-Style and Mortality in China: A Study of the Characteristics of 65 Chinese Counties* (Ithaca, N.Y.: Cornell University Press, 1990).

106 Best Stage 4 Foods: based on a list in Howard Markel, M.D., Jane A. Oski, M.D., Frank Oski, M.D., and Julia McMillan, M.D., *The Portable Pediatrician* (Philadelphia: Hanley & Belfus, 1992), p. 244.

107 substances that are not vitamins: Sharon Begley, "Beyond Vitamins," *Newsweek*, April 25, 1994, p. 45.

108 An-apple-a-day: David Schardt, "Phytochemicals: Plants Against Cancer," *Nutrition Action Healthletter*, April 1994.

108 consume . . . more potassium than sodium: National Academy of Sciences, *Recommended Daily Allowances* (Washington, D.C.: National Academy Press, 10th ed., 1989).

108 far more potassium: Richard D. Moore, M.D., Ph.D., and George D. Webb, Ph.D., *The K Factor* (New York: Pocket Books, 1986), pp. 30–33.

108 requirement of sodium: Lewis A. Barness, M.D., ed., *Pediatric Nutrition Handbook* (Elk Grove, Ill.: American Academy of Pediatrics, 1993).

Chapter 14
A Low-Fat Shopping Primer

111 hybrid fruits and vegetables: "New Fruits and Veggies for the '90s Cook," *U.S. News & World Report*, May 10, 1993.

111 new cucumber: Linda Negro, "What's Hot, What's Not in the World of Vegetables," Scripps Howard News Service, April 23, 1994.

112 little difference . . . between . . . white . . . and brown rice: Suzanne Havala, M.S., R.D., "Nutrition Hotline," *Vegetarian Journal*, March–April 1994, p. 2.

113 (such as Excalibur . . .): Marian Burros, "Eating Well: Beyond Teflon," *New York Times*, March 9, 1994, p. B6.

113 scraped with metal spoons: Kelly Costigan, "Melting Pots," *Health*, March–April 1994, pp. 91–93.

114 "Reduced-fat versions . . .": Skip Wollenberg, Associated Press, "Oreos, Ritz, Get the Reduced-Fat Treatment," *Denver Post*, March 30, 1994.

114 "-tos": Richard Gibson, *Wall Street Journal*, March 1, 1994.

114 InfoScan: Information Resources, Inc. 150 N. Clinton Street, Chicago, Ill. 60661; (312) 726-1221.

115 It isn't easy to find: Joseph C. Piscatella, *The Fat Tooth Fat Gram Counter* (New York: Workman, 1993), pp. 32–38.

117 Meatless burgers and franks: Michael DeBakey, Antonio Gotto, Lynne Scott, and John Foreyt, *The Living Heart Brand Name Shopper's Guide* (New York: Mastermedia Limited, 1993).

120 all packaged foods: ibid., pp. 78–93.

121 David Kessler said: Richard Gibson, "Label Law Stirs Up Food Companies," *Wall Street Journal*, June 2, 1993, p. B1.

123 "potential for concern": National Academy of Sciences, *Pesticides in the Diets of Infants and Children* (Washington, D.C.: National Academy Press), June 1993.

124 standards are adequate: personal communication from Cato Institute, Washington, D.C., phone (202) 842-0200.

124 linger in fish: Rachel Carson, *Silent Spring* (New York: Houghton Mifflin, 1962), pp. 129–52.

124 high levels of DDT: D. Steinman, *Environmental Toxicology and Chemistry*, vol. 8, no. 1 (1989).

124 Excess calories alone: personal communication from Dr. Ronald Hart, May 1994.

125 "vanishingly small": personal communication from Dr. Gladys Block, Department of Public Health, University of California at Berkeley.

126 Richard J. Jackson commented: John Hastings, "Do Pesticides on Fruits and Veggies Threaten Children?" *Health*, Sept. 1993, p. 12.

126 such as NutriClean: Christopher S. Kilham, *The Bread & Circus Whole Food Bible* (New York: Addison-Wesley, 1991), p. 19.

Chapter 15
Back Home, Getting Started

131 "quiet cooking": Robert James Waller, *The Bridges of Madison County* (New York: Warner Books, 1992), p. 54.

Chapter 16
When Children Eat Out

133 "drive-through window": personal communication from Dr. Peter Jones, 1991.

133 Meatless burgers: Jayne Hurley and Stephen Schmidt, "Meatless in Burgerland," *Nutrition Action Healthletter*, March 1994.

134 fettuccini Alfredo: Jayne Hurley and Bonnie Liebman, "When in Rome," *Nutrition Action Healthletter*, Jan.–Feb. 1994, pp. 6–7.

135 typical Mexican: ibid., July–Aug. 1994, pp. 4–7.

138 "doggie bag": Hope S. Warshaw, M.M.Sc., R.D., *Eat Out, Eat Right* (Chicago: Surrey Books, 1992), p. 8.

Chapter 17
School Lunch Programs

140 12 minutes: Marian Burros, "Eating Well," *New York Times*, Dec. 8, 1993.

141 taught to eat: Neal Barnard, M.D., *Food for Life* (New York: Harmony Books, 1993), p. xiv.

142 "They need the calcium . . .": Linda Castarone, "Moooove Over, Chocolate Milk," *Rocky Mountain News*, March 23, 1993.

142 "Fatalities, 70 percent": Rick Hampson, Associated Press, *Denver Post*, Oct. 20, 1993.

143 banded together: Dr. Earl Mindell, *Parents' Nutrition Bible* (Carson, Calif.: Hay House, 1992), p. 148.

144 New Orleans . . . survey: R. P. Farris, T. A. Nicklas, L. S. Webber, and G. S. Berenson, "Nutrient Contribution of the School Lunch Program: Implications for Healthy People 2000," *Journal of School Health*, vol. 62, no. 5 (May 1992), pp. 180–84.

145 ". . . french-fry deprivation": Laura Shapiro, "Fat Times at Ridgemont High," *Newsweek*, Nov. 8, 1993.

145 reported in 1993: R. C. Whitaker et al., *Journal of Pediatrics*, vol. 123 (1993), pp. 857–62.

146 LUNCHPOWER! M. P. Snyder, M. Story, and L. L. Trenkner, "Reducing Fat and Sodium in School Lunch Programs: The Lunchpower Intervention Study," *Journal of the American Diet Association*, vol. 92, no. 9 (Sept. 1992), pp. 1087–91.

146 intervention in New Orleans: M. L. Arbeit, C. C. Johnson, D. S. Mott, D. W. Harsha et al., "The Heart Smart Cardiovascular School Health Promotion: Behavior Correlates of Risk Factor Change," *Preventive Medicine*, vol. 21, no. 1 (Jan. 1992), pp. 18–32.

147 Jane L. Newmark: *Heart Healthy Lessons for Children* (Phoenix, Ariz.: Arizona Heart Institute and Foundation, 1991).

148 St. Martin Parish: personal communication from Ronald Chevalier, superintendent of schools, St. Martin Parish.

148 "Lunch at the Waldorf": personal communication from Andrea Huff.

148 to encourage healthful eating: personal communication from the Hearty School Lunch Program, American Heart Association.

148 Texas school districts: personal communication from Health Star, American Heart Association Texas Affiliate, 1615 Stemmons Freeway, Dallas, Tex. 75207

149 introduced legislation: personal communication from Patrick J. Leahy, United States Senate, Committee on Agriculture, Nutrition, and Forestry.

Chapter 18
The Childhood Beginnings of Heart Disease

153 "As a cardiologist": Greg Phillips, M.S., *The Think Light! Lowfat Living Plan* (Durango, Colo.: Speaking of Fitness, 1988), author quoting Dr. Steven Van Camp. Also personal communication from Dr. Van Camp.

154 Bogalusa Heart Study: G. Berenson et al., "Atherosclerosis of the Aorta and Cardiovascular Risk Factors in Persons Aged 6 to 30 Years and Studied at Necropsy (Bogalusa Heart Study)," *American Journal of Cardiology*, vol. 70 (1992), pp. 851–58.

154 "fatty streaks": W. P. Newman, W. Wattigney, and G. S. Berenson, "Autopsy Studies in United States Children and Adolescents," *Annals of the New York Academy of Science*, vol. 623 (1991), pp. 16–25.

154 evidence . . . not the first: R. L. Holman, H. C. McGill, Jr., J. P. Strong, and J. C. Geer, "The Natural History of Atherosclerosis: The Early Aortic Lesions as Seen in New Orleans in the Middle of the 20th Century," *American Journal of Pathology*, vol. 34 (1958), pp. 209–35.

155 in Europe as early as 1930: P. Zeek, "Juvenile Arteriosclerosis," *Archives of Pathology*, vol. 10 (1930), pp. 417–46.

155 More recent autopsy studies: H. C. Stary, "Evolution and Progression of Atherosclerotic Lesions in Coronary Arteries of Children and Young Adults," *Atherosclerosis*, vol. 9, suppl. 1 (1989), pp. 1-19–1-32; H. C. Stary, "The Sequence of Cell and Matrix Changes in Atherosclerotic Lesions of Coronary Arteries in the First 40 Years of Life," *European Heart Journal*, vol. 11, suppl. E (1990), pp. 3–19.

155 ". . . 3 years old": Paula Einhorn, M.D., and Basil Rifkind, M.D., editorial, *American Journal of Diseases of Childhood*, vol. 147 (April 1993), p. 373–75.

155 first report appeared: PDAY Research Group, "Relationship of Atherosclerosis in Young Men to Serum Lipoprotein Cholesterol Concentrations and Smoking: A Preliminary Report from the Pathobiological Determinants of Atherosclerosis in Youth (PDAY) Research Group," *JAMA*, vol. 264 (1990), pp. 3018–24.

155 group's latest report: PDAY Research Group, "Natural History of Aortic and Coronary Atherosclerotic Lesions in Youth," *Arteriosclerosis and Thrombosis*, vol. 13 (1993), pp. 1291–98.

156 1,017 medical students: M. J. Klag, D. E. Ford, L. A. Mead, J. He et al., "Serum Cholesterol in Young Men and Subsequent Cardiovascular Disease," *New England Journal of Medicine*, vol. 329, no. 2 (July 8, 1993), p. 138.

156 "killed in battle": J. P. Strong, "Coronary Atherosclerosis in Soldiers: A Clue to the Natural History of Atherosclerosis in the Young," *JAMA*, vol. 256 (1986), pp. 2863–66.

156 "Korean": W. F. Enos, R. H. Holmes, and J. Beyer, "Coronary Disease Among United States Soldiers Killed in Action in Korea: Preliminary Report," *JAMA*, vol. 152 (1953), pp. 1090–93.

156 "Vietnam wars": J. J. McNamara, M. A. Molot, J. F. Stremple, and R. T. Butting, "Coronary Artery Disease in Combat Casualties in Vietnam," *Jama*, vol. 216 (1971), pp. 1185–87.

156 "In the year 2030 . . . ": personal communication from Dr. Gerald Berenson.

157 Muscatine, Iowa, study: R. M. Lauer and W. R. Clarke, "Use of Cholesterol Measurements in Childhood for the Prediction of Adult Hypercholesterolemia: The Muscatine Study," *JAMA*, vol. 264, no. 23 (Dec. 19, 1990), pp. 3034–38.

157 disease *progresses:* Dean Ornish, M.D., letter to the editor, *JAMA*, vol. 267, no. 3 (Jan. 15, 1992), p. 362.

158 most notable: B. G. Brown, J. J. Alberts, L. D. Fisher et al., "Regression of Coronary Artery Disease as a Result of Intensive Lipid-lowering Therapy in Men with High Levels of Apolipoprotein B," *New England Journal of Medicine*, vol. 323 (1990), app. 1289–98.

158 1 child in 14,000: personal communication from Office of Public Health (DHH) Genetic Disease Program, New Orleans, La., June 23, 1994.

158 1 in 1,000 with deafness: Sherry Boschert, "Universal Screening for Hearing Loss in Newborns Stalled by Cost Controversy," *Pediatric News*, March 1994, p. 16.

158 (20 million): personal communication from AHA President Suzanne Oparil, M.D.

158 ". . . next generation of heart attacks": Robert A. Barnett, "Cholesterol Testing of Kids Questioned," *Denver Post*, March 20, 1994, pp. 1, 3-E.

158 My position: Charles Attwood, M.D., *Pediatric Management*, November 1991.

159 "Why create an impression . . .": Katarzyna Wandycz, "Too Young to Diet," *Forbes*, Aug. 16, 1993.

159 just like their parents: National Center for Health Statistics, Hyattsville, Md., Hospital Discharge Survey, August 1988.

159 299 families: R. Garcia and D. Moodie, "Routine Cholesterol Surveillance in Children," *Pediatrics*, vol. 84, no. 5 (Nov. 1989), pp. 751–55.

160 Among 1,005 children: T. C. Griffin, K. K. Christoffel, H. J. Binns, and P. A. McGuire, "Family History Evaluation as a Predictive Screen for Childhood Hypercholesterolemia," *Pediatrics*, vol. 84, no. 2 (Aug. 1989), pp. 365–73.

160 Pam Mycoskie: Marty Meitus, "Buttering Up to Low-Fat Ways," *Rocky Mountain News*, March 30, 1994.

161 only three months: E. S. Quivers, D. J. Driscoll, C. D. Garvey, A. M. Harris et al., "Variability in Response to a Low-Fat, Low-Cholesterol Diet in Children with Elevated Low-Density Lipoprotein Cholesterol Levels," *Pediatrics*, no. 5, pt. 1 (May 1992), pp. 925–29.

161 (KYB) Study: H. J. Walter, A. Hofman, R. D. Vaughan, and E. L. Wynder, "Modification of Risk Factors for Coronary Heart Disease," *New England Journal of Medicine*, vol. 318 (1988), pp. 1096–1100.

162 children in Baltimore: K. Stewart et al., "The Three-Year Evaluation of FRESH (Food Re-education for Elementary School Health): A Nutrition-Focused School-Based Heart Health Program," *Circulation*, vol. 4 (1993), pp. 11–14.

162 "cook-off": K. M. Gans, S. Levin, T. Lasater et al., "Heart Healthy Cook-offs in Home Economics Classes: An Evaluation with Junior High School Students," *Journal of School Health*, vol. 60, no. 3 (March 1990), pp. 99–101.

163 Japanese diet . . . has become Westernized: K. Tanaka, "Lessons in Prevention of Atherosclerosis Learned from Recent Studies of Japanese Youth, *Annals of the New York Academy of Sciences*, vol. 598 (1990), pp. 398–409.

163 urban Japanese children: Marian Burros "Eating Well," *New York Times*, April 13, 1994, p. B10.

164 1 month to 39 years: K. Tanaka et al., "A Nation-wide Study of Atherosclerosis in Infants, Children, and Young Adults in Japan," *Atherosclerosis*, vol. 72 (1988), pp. 143–56.

164 ". . . clear-cut need for guidelines . . .": I. A. Kashani and P. R. Nader, "The Role of the Pediatrician in the Prevention of Coronary Heart Disease in Childhood," *Japanese Heart Journal*, vol. 27, no. 6 (Nov. 1986), pp. 911–22.

164 more than 1,000 restaurants: Marian Burros, "Eating Well," *New York Times*, April 13, 1994, p. B10.

164 experiencing a sharp increase: "Epidemiology of Coronary Arterial Disease in the Chinese," *International Journal of Cardiology*, vol. 24 (1989), pp. 83–93.

165 urban Chinese population: Jan Wong, "Hunger to Obesity: Chinese Fighting Battle of the Bulge," *Rocky Mountain News*, March 17, 1994, p. 36A.

165 city-state: K. Hughes, P. Yeo, K. Lun et al., "Ischaemic Heart Disease and Its Risk Factors in Singapore in Comparison with Other Countries," *Annals Academy of Medicine*, vol. 18, no. 3 (May 1989), pp. 245–49.

165 among Singaporian children: K. Hughes, ibid., p. 245.

165 these 6,500 Chinese: J. Chen, T. C. Campbell, J. Li, and R. Peto, *Diet, Life-Style and Mortality in China* (Ithaca, N.Y.: Cornell University Press, 1990).

166 *155 times higher:* Jane Brody, "Hugh Study of Diet Indicts Fat and Meat," *New York Times*, May 8, 1990, section C.

167 in the two communities: W. Freeman, D. C. Weir, J. E. Whitehead, D. I. Rogers et al., "Association Between Risk Factors for Coronary Heart Disease in School-boys and Adult Mortality Rates in the Same Localities," *Archives of Diseases of Childhood*, vol. 65, no. 1 (1990), pp. 78–83.

167 *children ages 1 to 5:* A. Angelini, G. Thiene, C. Frescura, and G. Baroldi, "Coronary Arterial Wall and Atherosclerosis in Youth (1–20 Years): A Histologic Study in a Northern Italian Population," *International Journal of Cardiology*, vol. 28, no. 3 (Sept. 1990), pp. 361–70.

167 city of Milan: M. Giovannini, R. Bellu, M. T. Ortisi et al., "Cholesterol and Lipoprotein Levels in Milanese Children: Relation to Nutritional and Familial Factors," *Journal of the American College of Nutrition*, vol. 11, suppl. (June 1992), pp. 28S–31S.

168 multinational studies: E. L. Wynder et al., "Screening for Risk Factors for Chronic Disease in Children from Fifteen Countries," *Preventive Medicine*, vol. 10 (1981), pp. 121–32; J. T. Knuiman et al., "Serum Total and High-Density Lipoprotein Cholesterol Concentrations in Rural and Urban Boys from 16 Countries," *Atherosclerosis*, vol. 36 (1980), pp. 529–37.

168 serum-cholesterol levels . . . decreased: J. Viikari, H. K. Akerblom, L. Rasanen, M. Kalavainen, and O. Pietarinen, "Cardiovascular Risk in Young Finns: Experiences from the Finnish Multicentre Study Regarding the Prevention of Coronary Heart Disease," *Acta Paediatricia Scandinavia*, vol. 365, suppl. (1990), pp. 13–19.

168 private and public schools: S. Mendoza, G. Contreras, E. Ineichen, M. Fernandez et al., "Lipids and Lipoproteins in Venezuelan and American Schoolchildren: Within and Cross-cultural Comparisons," *Pediatric Research*, vol. 14, no. 4, pt. 1 (April 1980), pp. 272–77.

169 976 black subjects: K. Steyn, M. L. Langenhoven, G. Joubert, D. O. Chalton et

al., "The Relationship Between Dietary Factors and Serum Cholesterol Values in the Coloured Population of the Cape Peninsula," *Southern African Medical Journal*, vol. 78, no. 2 (July 21, 1990), pp. 63–67.

169 Indian, colored, and white: Y. K. Seedat, F. G. Mayet, G. H. Latiff, and G. Joubert, "Risk Factors and Coronary Heart Disease in Durban Blacks—the Missing Links," *Southern African Medical Journal*, vol. 82, no. 4 (Oct. 1992), pp. 251–56.

170 against all consumption of cow's milk: Marian Burros, "Eating Well," *New York Times*, September 30, 1992, p. B5.

170 ". . . designed for calves . . .": David Stipp, "Doctor Spock Adds Clout to Warning About Cow's Milk," *Wall Street Journal*, Sept. 30, 1992.

170 "nutritional terrorism . . .": Marian Burros, "Eating Well," *New York Times*, Sept. 30, 1992, p. B5.

171 principal author of: Suzanne Havala and Johanna Dwyer, "Position of the American Dietetic Association: Vegetarian Diets," *Journal of the American Dietetic Association*, vol. 93 (1993), pp. 1317–19. Also personal communication from Ms. Havala.

Chapter 19
Summit in the Desert

173 ambitious project: 1st National Conference on the Elimination of Coronary Artery Disease, Loew's Ventana Canyon Resort, Tucson, Ariz., Oct. 3–4, 1991, Caldwell B. Esselstyn Foundation, 1201 Troy-Schenectady Road, Latham, N.Y. 12110.

176 can actually reverse: D. Ornish et al., "Can Lifestyle Changes Reverse Coronary Heart Disease?," *Lancet*, vol. 336 (1990), pp. 129–33.

176 now cover expenses: Molly O'Neill, "Unusual Heart Therapy Wins Coverage from Large Insurer," *New York Times*, July 28, 1993, p. A1.

178 mice . . . just died suddenly: personal communication from Dr. Ronald Hart.

178 greatly reduced animal protein: personal communication from Dr. T. Colin Campbell.

178 Roy Walford: William M. Bortz II, M.D., *We Live Too Short and Diet Too Long* (New York: Bantam, Books, 1991), p. 38.

180 consensus . . . endorsed and signed: personal communication from Caldwell B. Esselstyn, Jr., M.D.

Chapter 20
How You're Misinformed

182 "gains . . . are modest": J. Tsevat, M. Weinstein, L. Williams et al., "Expected Gains in Life Expectancy from Various Coronary Heart Disease Risk Factor Modifications," *Circulation*, vol. 83 (1991), pp. 1194–1201.

183 "talk healthy diets . . .": "Heart Doctors Feast on Fries," *Advocate* (Baton Rouge, La.), Nov. 10, 1993.

184 life-style habits: L. Breslow and N. Breslow, "Health Practices and Disability:

Some Evidence from Alameda County," *Preventive Medicine*, vol. 22, no. 1 (Jan. 1993), pp. 86–95.

185 "Strict adherence . . .": F. Lifshitz, "Children on Adult Diets: Is It Harmful? Is It Healthy?," *Journal of the American College of Nutrition*, vol. 11, Suppl. (June 1992), pp. 84S–90S.

186 poor, malnourished: T. Nicklas, L. Webber, M. Koschak, and G. Berenson, "Nutritional Adequacy of Lowfat Intakes for Children," *Pediatrics*, vol. 89, no. 2, p. 221–28.

186 B-vitamin deficiencies: C. S. Lo, "Riboflavin Status of Adolescent Southern Chinese," *Human Nutrition: Clinical Nutrition*, vol. 39C, no. 4 (July 1985), pp. 297–301; T. A. Brun, J. Chen, T. C. Campbell et al., "Urinary Riboflavin Excretion After a Load Test in Rural China as a Measure of Possible Riboflavin Deficiency," *European Journal of Clinical Nutrition*, vol. 44 (1990), pp. 195–206.

186 reduction in cholesterol: D. Hunninghake et al., "The Efficacy of Intense Dietary Therapy Alone, or Combined with Lovastatin in the Outpatient with Hypercholesterolemia," *New England Journal of Medicine*, vol. 328 (March 1993), pp. 1213–19.

187 eleventh annual study: "Update: Eleventh Supplement PREVENTION PROGRAM PROFILES," *Prevention*, January 1994, pp. 49–51.

187 a turn for the worse: "Americans Continue to Put On Yet More Weight," Harris Poll, 1994, #26, Louis Harris & Associates, 630 Fifth Avenue, New York, N.Y.; (212) 698-9697.

187 National Heart, Lung, and Blood Institute: D. Jacobs, H. Blackburn, D. Reed et al., "Report on the Conference on Low Blood Cholesterol: Mortality Associations," *Circulation*, vol. 86, no. 3 (Sept. 1992), pp. 1046–60.

187 12-year study: J. D. Neaton, H. Blackburn, D. Jacobs, L. Kuller et al., "Serum Cholesterol Level and Mortality Findings for Men Screened in the Multiple Risk Factor Intervention Trial Research Group," *Archives of Internal Medicine*, vol. 153, no. 10 (May 24, 1992), pp. 1268–71.

188 Framingham Study: D. Ornish, letter to the editor, *Lancet*, Sept. 22, 1990, pp. 741–42.

188 MRFIT trials: "Risk Factor Changes and Mortality Results," *JAMA*, vol. 248 (Sept. 1982), pp. 1465–77.

188 cholesterol level was a "marker": J. Stamler and J. Neaton, "Benefits of Lower Cholesterol," *Scientific American Science Medicine*, vol. 1, no. 2 (May–June 1994), pp. 28–37.

188 20-year-olds: M. J. Flag, D. E. Ford, L. A. Mead, J. He et al., "Serum Cholesterol in Young Men and Subsequent Cardiovascular Disease, *New England Journal of Medicine*, vol. 329, no. 2 (July 8, 1993), p. 138.

189 no longer be checked in women: S. Hulley, J. M. B. Walsh, and T. B. Newman, "Health Policy on Blood Cholesterol: Time to Change Directions," *Circulation*, vol. 86 (1992), pp. 1026–29.

189 women are more likely to die: *Daily Advertiser*, Lafayette, La., quoting Dr. Richard Beeker, who was interviewed by *American Health*, April 29, 1991, p. D1.

189 abandon all cholesterol testing: S. Hulley, T. Newman, D. Grady et al., "Should We Be Measuring Blood Cholesterol Levels in Young Adults?," *JAMA*, vol. 269, no. 11 (March 17, 1993), p. 1416.

189 ". . . not at kids": Robert A. Barnett, "Cholesterol Testing of Kids Questioned," *Denver Post*, March 20, 1994, pp. 1E–3E.

190 die of other diseases: Rose G. and M. Shipley, "Effects of Coronary Risk Reduction on the Pattern of Mortality," *Lancet*, vol. 335, no. 8684 (Feb. 3, 1990), pp. 275–77.

190 £12,400: I. S. Kristiansen, A. E. Eggen, and D. S. Thelle, "Cost Effectiveness of Incremental Programmes for Lowering Serum Cholesterol Concentration: Is Individual Intervention Worth While?," *British Medical Journal*, vol. 302, no. 6785 (May 11, 1991), pp. 1119–22.

191 cost $1 million: J. Walsh and T. B. Newman, "Cholesterol Screening in Young Adults," *JAMA*, vol. 270, no. 13 (Oct. 6, 1993), pp. 1546–47.

191 10-year-old boys: The Harvard Lifesaving Study, 1994. Unpublished.

191 $40 per week: Neal Barnard, M.D., *Food for Life* (New York: Harmony Books, 1993), p. xii.

191 $1,500 per year: Reed Mangels, Ph.D., *Vegetarian Journal*, March–April 1994, p. 2.

192 "If you love rich desserts . . . ": William A. Nolen, M.D., *Crisis Time! Love, Marriage and the Male at Midlife* (New York: Dodd, Mead, 1984), 144–46.

193 nutritional backlash: Dr. Susan Calvert Finn, American Dietetic Association, in Howard Goldberg, Associated Press, *Denver Post*, October 20, 1993, p. 14A.

193 toward high-fat foods: personal communication from Martin Root, Cornell University, October 1993.

Recommended Reading

General Interest and Reference

Bailey, Covert. *The New Fit or Fat.* Boston: Houghton Mifflin, 1991.

Barnard, Neal, M.D., with recipes by Jennifer Raymond. *Food for Life: How the New Four Food Groups Can Save Your Life.* New York: Harmony Books, 1993

Campbell, Susan and Todd Winant. *Healthy School Lunch Action Guide.* EarthSave (706 Frederick Street, Santa Cruz, CA 95062).

DeBakey, Michael E., Antonio M. Gotto, Jr., Lynne W. Scott, and John P. Foreyt. *The Living Heart Brand Name Shopper's Guide.* New York: Mastermedia, 1993.

———. *The Living Heart Diet.* New York: Raven, 1984.

Goor, Ron, and Nancy Goor. *Eater's Choice: A Food Lover's Guide to Lower Cholesterol.* New York: Houghton Mifflin, 1992.

Gross, Joy. *Raising Your Family Naturally.* New York: Lyle Stuart, Inc., 1983.

Havala, Suzanne, M.S., R.D., and Mary Clifford, R.D. *Simple, Lowfat, and Vegetarian: Unbelievably Easy Ways to Reduce the Fat in Your Meals.* Vegetarian Resource Group (P.O. Box 1463, Baltimore, Md. 21203), 1994.

Heart-Healthy Lessons for Children. Phoenix, Ariz.: Arizona Heart Institute and Foundation, 1991.

Kilham, Christopher. *The Bread and Circus Whole Food Bible.* New York: Addison-Wesley, 1991.

Klaper, Michael, M.D. *Pregnancy, Children, and the Vegan Diet.* Paia, Hawaii: Gentle World, 1987. (Available from the American Vegan Society, 501 Old Harding Highway, Malaga, N.J. 08328)

Kwiterovick, Peter O., Jr., M.D. *The Johns Hopkins Complete Guide for Preventing and Reversing Heart Disease.* Rocklin, Calif.: Prima Publishing, 1993.

La Leche League International. *The Womanly Art of Breastfeeding.* New York: NAL/ Dutton, 1991.

Mangels, Reed, Ph.D., R.D. *Vegan Diet During Pregnancy, Lactation, and Childhood* (article reprint, 16 pgs.). Vegetarian Resource Group (P.O. Box 1463, Baltimore, Md. 21203), 1991.

McDougall, John, M.D., and Mary A. McDougall. *The McDougall Plan*. Hampton, N.J.: New Win, 1985.

Moran, Victoria. *Get the Fat Out: 501 Simple Ways to Cut the Fat in Any Diet*. New York: Crown Trade Paperbacks, 1994.

National Research Council. *Recommended Dietary Allowances,* 10th edition. Washington, D.C.: National Academy Press, 1989.

Ornish, Dean, M.D. *Dr. Dean Ornish's Program for Reversing Heart Disease*. New York: Random House, 1990.

Robbins, John. *May All Be Fed*. New York: Morrow, 1992.

Simone, Charles B., M.D. *Cancer and Nutrition: A Ten-Point Plan to Reduce Your Risk of Getting Cancer*. Garden City Park, N.Y.: Avery Publishing Group, 1992.

Warshaw, Hope S. *Eat Out, Eat Right*. Chicago: Surrey Books, 1992.

The Wellness Encyclopedia of Food and Nutrition. University of California at Berkeley. New York: Rebus, 1992.

Woteki, Catherine E., Ph.D., and Paul R. Thomas, Ed.D., eds. *Eat for Life*. Washington, D.C.: National Academy Press, 1992. New York: HarperPerennial, 1993.

Yntema, Sharon. *Vegetarian Baby*. Ithaca, N.Y.: McBooks Press, 1980.

———. *Vegetarian Children*. Ithaca, N.Y.: McBooks Press, 1987.

Low-Fat Cookbooks

Ballantyne, Penny, and Maureen Egan. *Low Salt, Low Sugar, Low Fat Desserts*. San Leandro, Calif.: Bristol, 1988.

Bluestein, Barry, and Kevin Morrissey. *The 99% Fat-Free Cookbook*. New York: Doubleday, 1994.

Daley, Rosie. *In the Kitchen with Rosie*. New York: Knopf, 1994.

Dunn, S. *Bearly Any Fat*. Iowa Falls, Iowa: General Publishing and Binding, 1994.

Gotto, Antonio M., Jr., M.D. *The Living Heart Cookbook*. New York: Fireside, 1991.

Levy, Faye. *Faye Levy's International Vegetable Cookbook*. New York: Warner Books, 1994.

McDougall, John, M.D., and Mary A. McDougall. *The New McDougall Cookbook*. New York: NAL/Dutton, 1993.

Moquette-Magee, Elaine, M.P.H., R.D. *200 Kid-Tested Ways to Lower the Fat in Your Child's Favorite Foods*. Minneapolis, Minn.: Chronimed Publishing, 1993.

Mycoskie, Pam. *Butter Busters, the Cookbook*. New York: Warner Books, 1994.

Piscatella, Joseph C. *Controlling Your Fat Tooth*. New York: Workman Publishing, 1991.

Shandler, Michael, and Nina Shandler. *The Complete Guide and Cookbook to Raising Your Child as a Vegetarian*. New York: Schocken, 1987.

Sunset Low-Fat Cookbook. Menlo Park, Calif.: Sunset, 1993.

Wagner, Lindsay, and Ariane Spade. *The High Road to Health: A Vegetarian Cookbook*. New York: Prentice-Hall, 1990.

The Wellness Lowfat Cookbook. University of California at Berkeley. New York: Rebus, 1993.

Williams, Jacqueline, and Goldie Silverman. *No Salt, No Sugar, No Fat Cookbook*. San Leandro, Calif.: Bristol, 1993.

Newsletters

Lifeline
Lifestyle Medicine Institute
Better Health
P.O. Box 1761
Loma Linda, Calif. 92354

Nutrition Action Healthletter
Center for Science in the Public Interest
1875 Connecticut Ave., N.W., Suite 300
Washington, D.C. 20009-5728

The Nutrition Advocate
Senior Editor T. Colin Campbell, Ph.D.,
P.O. Box 4716
Ithaca, N.Y. 14852

Tufts University Diet & Nutrition Letter
53 Park Place
New York, N.Y. 10007

University of California at Berkeley Wellness Letter
P.O. Box 420148
Palm Coast, Fla. 32142

The University of Texas–Houston Health Science Center Lifetime Health Letter
7000 Fannin
Houston, Tex. 77030

Index

Adipose tissue, 32
Aerobic exercise, 31
Africans, xxi, 169
After-school habits, 22
Agricultural Revolution, 30
Airline food, 137–38
Alabaster, Dr. Oliver, 44, 47
Alar, 122, 125
Alcoholism, 187–88
Allergies and dairy products, 63, 64, 76, 171
Allyl sulfides, 107
American Academy of Pediatrics (AAP), xx, 83, 150
   cholesterol levels set by, 5, 8, 12–13, 156–60, 171
   Committee on Nutrition, 13, 64, 108, 159, 170
   inadequate dietary guidelines of, xxv–xxvi
   on milk, 64
American Airlines, 137
American Cancer Society, 60, 150
American Health Foundation, 26, 44, 52, 162
American Heart Association (AHA), xxiv, xxvii, 11, 103, 182, 183
   on beans, 60
   cholesterol levels and, 4, 5, 156–58
   dietary guidelines of, xxvi, xxviii, 91, 144, 171, 172, 175–77
   iron, LDL levels and, 58
   school lunches and, 144, 148–49
   Step I diet, 42–43
   Step II diet, 186
"Americanized diet," xvii, xxi–xxiii, 4, 96, 180
   in Africa, 169
   in Asia, 163–66
   changes in, 59, 61
   in England, 166–67
   in Italy, 167–68
   obesity and, 30–31
   saturated fats in, 17
   in South America, 168–69
   vitamins, minerals and, 70–71
American Journal of Cardiology, 5, 154
American Journal of Clinical Nutrition, 67
American Journal of Medicine, 184
American School Food Service Association, 141
Ames, Dr. Bruce, 125–26
Amino acids, 58–59
Animal protein, *see* Meat
Annals of Internal Medicine, 19
Antioxidants, 72–73
Antioxidant Vitamin Counter, The (Natow and Heslin), 70
Apple Crisp, 243
Applesauce Muffins, 244
Archives of Internal Medicine, 187–89
Arizona Heart Institute, 147–48
Arteriosclerosis, 184
"Artificial fat," 37
Asians, 19–20
Associated Press, 114, 142, 183

Atherosclerosis, xxv, 164
Atlantic, The, 97, 98
Avocados, 110

Babies, feeding, 200–2
"Bad cholesterol," 14–15
"Balanced meal," 210
Baltimore school lunches, 140
Baltimore Sun, 93
Banana:
  "Ice Cream," 223–24
  -Oat Muffins, 246
  Pancakes, 225–26
  Smoothies, 227
Bantus, 66
Barbara's Mini Whole Wheat Pretzels,
  115
Barga, Steven, 142
Barnard, Dr. Neal, 7, 29, 38, 46–47,
  66, 102, 141, 170, 191
Basic Banana Smoothie, 227
Baskin Robbins, 165
Baylor University, xxvii, 44, 133
Beans:
  protein from, 56–60, 69
  shopping for, 113
Beans, Refried, 237–38
Beef industry, xxvi, xxix, xxx, 55–56,
  96
Benadryl, 24
Berenson, Dr. Gerald, 46, 50, 154,
  156, 157, 158, 173, 177
Berry Smoothie, Banana-, 227
Beta-carotene, 71, 72, 80, 81, 111
  supplements of, 19
"Better Nutrition and Health for Chil-
  dren Act of 1994," 149–50
Betts, George Herbert, vi
Beyond Beef (Rifkin), 61
Bible, 83
Biotin, 75–76
Birch, Dr. Leann, 37
Bismark, Prince Otto von, 95
Block, Dr. Gladys, 125
Blankenhorn, Dr. David, 46
Blood pressure, 27
Blueberry:
  "Ice Cream," 224
  Shake, 228
Bogalusa Heart Study, 9, 23, 26, 46,
  50, 154–56
Bortz, Dr. Walter, 21, 183–84
Boyle, Dr. Peter, xxii
Boyle, T. Coraghessan, 55

Bran, 93
Brandeis University, 48
Bread, 112
  Corn, 249
Breakfast recipes, 223–29
Breast cancer, xxii–xxiii, 56, 166, 184
Breslow, Dr. Lester, 184
Bridges of Madison County, The (Wal-
  ler), 131
Brigham Young University, 24
"Broccoflower," 111
Brody, Jane, 66, 125
Brown, Dr. B. G., 158
Buffon, Charles, 88
Burger King, 52
Burkitt, Dr. Denis, xxiv
Bushmen, 8, 40
Butler, Samuel, 172
Butter Busters: The Cookbook (Mycos-
  kie), 160

Cake:
  Chocolate-Brownie, 247
  Pineapple Upside-Down, 245
Calcium, 171
  bone density and, 65
  myth concerning, 62–69
  sources of, 66–68
Caldwell B. Esselstyn Foundation, 173
Calories, 32–34, 44, 70
  calcium and, 67–68
  low-fat snacks and, 94
  vegetarian diets and, 85–86
Campbell, Dr. T. Colin, xxviii–xxix, 43,
  47, 88, 102, 166, 173, 178–79
Cancer, xxviii, 11, 166, 179
  animal protein and, 56–57
  antioxidants and, 72
  high-fat diet and, xxi–xxiv
  misinformation about, 184, 187–88
  pesticides and, 122–26
  phytochemicals and, 107–8
  see also specific types of cancer
Canola oil, 18, 94, 113
Cara-Bunch, 111
Carbohydrates, 32
  calories and, 32–34
  complex, 31–32, 88
Cardiology, 188
Carl's Jr., 52
Carroll, Lewis, 36
Carson, Rachel, 124
Castelli, Dr. William, 6–7, 79, 97, 173,
  177

Cato Institute, 124
Causes of death, leading, xx, 49
Center for Epidemiological Research in Southern Africa, 169
Center for Science in the Public Interest, 80, 94, 114, 133–34, 150
Centers for Disease Control and Prevention (CDC), xxvi, 26
  Division of Nutrition, 85
Cereals, shopping for, 111–12
Chambrin, Pierre, 89–90
Chandler Arizona Food Service, 147–148
Cheese, 63
Chef's Expressions Catering, 93
Chevalier, Roland, 148
Chicago Heart Association, 188
Chicken, 115, 116
Child and Adolescent Trial for Cardiovascular Health (CATCH 1990), 141
Childhood beginnings of disease, 153–71
  Bogalusa Heart Study, 154–56
  dietary intervention, 160–62
  educational intervention, 161–62
  family history and, 159–60
  in foreign countries, *see* International high-fat life-style
  identifying those at risk, 156–57
  Johns Hopkins Young Adult Study, 156
  Muscatine, Iowa, study, 157–58
  universal cholesterol testing and, 158–59
Child Nutrition Act of 1966, 150
Children's Defense Fund, 150
Children's Treatment Panel, 8
Chili, Vegetarian, 242
China, xxi, 8, 9, 15, 19–20, 56, 59, 65–66, 73, 75, 81, 88, 105, 165–66, 175–76, 177, 185–88
China Health Study, xxviii, xxix, 19, 66, 73, 88, 165–66, 175
Chinese restaurants, 135
Chinese University of Hong Kong, 164
Chlorogenic acid, 107
Chocolate-Brownie Cake, 247
Chocolate-Chip Cranberry Cookies, 248
Cholesterol, xx
  animal protein and, 56

autopsy data and, 3, 12, 97, 154–156, 164, 167
cost-effectiveness of reducing, 190–191
dairy products and, 63, 65
described, 14–15
foods high in, 90–91
growth and, 87
inadequate "official" dietary guidelines and, xxv–xxviii
level of:
  adult risk, 8
  checking all family members, 12–13
  in children, 3–4, 12–13
  controlling high, 16–17
  guidelines for children's, 9, 12–13
  heart-disease risk and, 9–10
  ideal, 9
  lowering, 19, 42, 44, 190–91
  over 150, 5–8
  risk of low, 187–90
  what's high, what's not, 8
Mediterranean or Asian way, 19–20
misinformation about, *see* Misinformation
myth concerning, 3–20
pediatricians and, 12–13
power of prevention, 10–11
saturated fat and, 16–19
statistics concerning, 4, 12
testing for, 14
  abandonment of, 189–90
see also Childhood beginnings of disease
"Cholesterol Myth, The," 97
Chowder, Potato-Corn, 237
Circulation, 58, 182, 187–89
Cleveland Clinic, 159, 172, 173
Clinton, Bill, 53, 150
Clinton, Hillary Rodham, 53, 89–90, 150
Coconut oil, 17, 93–94
Coconuts, 110
Colon cancer, 20, 25, 56, 57
  fiber and, 60, 107
Columbia University, 19
Commercials, TV, 22
Condiments, 92–93
Conflicting advice, 95–98
  certified facts, 96–97
  proof of, 97–98
  "planned" confusion, 96
Conner, Dr. William, 29

Constipation, 11
Contemporary Pediatrics, xxx
Conti, Dr. C. Richard, 22
Cookies, 93, 94
  Chocolate-Chip Cranberry, 248
  Gingerbread, 250–51
  "Mud," 251–52
Corn Bread, 249
Corn Chowder, Potato-, 237
Cornell University, xxvii, 102, 126,
    165, 178, 193
Corn oil, 18
Coronary heart (artery) disease:
  antioxidants and, 72
  bypass surgery for, 10–11
  cause of, xx, 5
  children's cholesterol levels and, 4
  costs of, xxiv, 11
  culture and, 20
  early appearance of, xix–xxi
  inadequate "official" dietary guide-
    lines and, xxiv–xxx, 44
  iron levels and, 58
  misinformation about, *see*
    Misinformation
  as number-one cause of death, xxi,
    27
  prevention of, xxi
  progression of, 44
  reversing, 175–77
  risk factors for developing, 5–6
    animal protein and, 56
    cholesterol levels and, 9–10, 49
  see also Childhood beginnings of
    disease
Cranberry Cookies, Chocolate-Chip,
    248
Crete, 20
Crisis Time! (Nolen), 192
Cucumbers, 111
Current Opinion in Pediatrics, xxxi
Cusiak, Neil, 27

Dairy industry, xxvi–xxvii, xxix, xxx,
    53, 62, 67, 96
Dairy products, xxvi–xxvii, 118
  coronary artery disease conference
    and, 177–78
  as high-fat food, 91, 170
  see also Milk
Dartmouth Medical School, 73
DDT, 124
DeBakey, Dr. Michael, 135
Delta Airlines, 137

Denver Post, 158, 186, 189
Denver school lunches, 142
Designs for Education, 142
Dessert and bread recipes, 243–52
Diabetes, xxiv, xxviii, 6, 11
  milk and, 63
  obesity and, 28–29
Diehl, Dr. Hans, xxiii, 7
Diet, xvii
  ideal, *see* Ideal diet
  misinformation about, *see*
    Misinformation
  "moderate," 101, 185
  return to high-fat, 183–87, 193
Diet and Health Report, 47
Dietary fat, 32–34
  token reductions in, *see* Token re-
    ductions of dietary fat
  see also High-fat foods
Dietary Intervention Study in Children
    (DISC), 86
Diethrich, Dr. Ted, 147
Diet, Nutrition, and Cancer, 57
Diseases of nutritional extravagance,
    xxviii, xxix, 61, 180
Diseases of poverty, xxix
Dodge, Dr. Harold T., 173
Domino's Pizza, 90
Dosch, Dr. Hans-Michael, 63
"Dr. Attwood's Low-Fat Guidelines,"
    128–29
*Dr. Dean Ornish's Program for Re-
    versing Heart Disease* (Ornish),
    34, 176
Dr. Spock's Baby and Child Care
    (Spock), 23, 37–38
Du Pont Silverstone, 113
Dwyer, Dr. Johanna, 71, 75

East Birmingham Hospital, 166–67
Eat for Life, xxi
Eating extremes, 206–10
Eating out, 133–38
  airline food, 137–38
  Chinese food, 135
  condiments, 135–36
  fast food, 133
  hotel breakfast, 136–37
  Italian food, 134
  Mexican food, 135
  salad bars, 136
Eat More, Weigh Less (Ornish), 34,
    176
Eaton, S. Boyd, 29–30

Eat Out, Eat Right (Warshaw), 138
Edwards, Jerry, 93
Eggplant Lasagna, Super-Saucy, 238–239
Eggs, 17, 53, 118
    fat and, 91
Egg substitutes, 91, 118
Elizabeth, 27–28
Emory University, 39
Empty calories, 32
Endosulfan, 122–23
England, 4, 65, 166–67
Enterostatin, 40
Eskimos, 66
Espy, Mike, 141
Esselstyn, Dr. Caldwell B., Jr., 172, 173, 179
Esselstyn, Dr. Caldwell Blakeman, 173
Essential amino acids, 58–59
Estrogen, 123
Excalibur, 113, 114
Exercise, 31–32, 207
"Expected Gains in Life Expectancy from Various Coronary Heart Disease Risk Factor Modifications," 182–83

Family Circle, 72, 135
Family dietary habits, 13–14, 26–29
Family history, 159–60
"Family plan," 131–32
Fanfare, 111
Farm Study, 85–86
Fast food, 50–53, 133, 164, 165, 183
Fat cells:
    genetics and, 32
    permanent, 25–26, 35
    storage in, 32–34
Fat-craving genes, 39–40
"Fat habit," xxvii–xxviii
"Fat taste," xxvii, 28
    chemical shortcut to tame, 40
    genes for, 39–40
    ideal diet and, 104, 105, 109
    learning and unlearning the, 37–38
    mechanics of, 37
    myth concerning, 36–40
    taming the, 38–39
    taste buds and, 36–37
"Fatty streaks," 154–56, 164
Federal government, xxix–xxx
Fiber, 60, 82
    Stage 4 diet and, 106–7
Fig Newtons, 94

Finland, 4, 43, 73, 168
Finn, Dr. Susan Calvert, 193
First National Cholesterol Conference, xxv, xxvi, 176
First National Conference on the Elimination of Coronary Artery Disease, 157, 172–80
    China Health Study and, 175
    consensus at, 175, 179–80
    dairy products and, 177–78
    Framingham Study and, 177
    life span and, 178–79
    panel members, 173–74
    reversing coronary disease, 175–77
Fish, 115, 116
    DDT and, 124
Fish oil, 19
FitFoods Fat Free, 115
Flavonoids, 108
"Flywheel effect," 31
Folic acid, 75, 111
Food and Agriculture Organization, 124
Food and Drug Administration (FDA), 75, 81, 113
    pesticides and, 123–24
Food for Life (Barnard), 38, 141
Food labels, 120–22
Food Marketing Institute, 62–63
Food Research and Action Center, 150
Food-smart family, 210–16
Four Food Groups, 204–5
    New, 198–99
Framingham Study, 6, 9, 79, 177, 188
France, 20, 30
Franklin, Benjamin, 181
Fred Hutchinson Cancer Research Center, 38
Friedman, Dr., 84
Fries, Dr. James F., 173
Frito-Lay, 114–15
Frozen products, 111
Fruit-Juice Smoothies and Shakes, 227–28
Fruits, 80–81
    cleaning, 126–27
    pesticides and, 122–26
    shopping for, 110–12

Galanin, 40
Garcia, Dr. Richard E., 159
Garden-Mexi, 104, 117
Garden-Sausage, 104, 117
Garden-Veggie, 104, 117, 133

Garlic, 19
Garrison, W. L., 101–2
Genetics:
    fat cells and, 32
    fat craving and, 39–40
    obesity and, 28–29
    produce and, 111
George Washington University, xxix,
        44, 102, 170, 191
Getting started, 128–32
Getting Thin (Mirkin), 42
Gibbons, Barry, 52
Gingerbread Cookies, 250–51
Goldberg, Dr., 84
"Gold-standard" diet, 108–9
"Good cholesterol," 14–15
Government dietary guidelines, xxiv–
        xxx
    fears of discouraging the public
        and, 43–49
Grains, 111
Granola, 92
Granola, Low-Fat, 229
Grape-Nuts, 92
Gray, Thomas, 1
Great Atlantic & Pacific Tea Co., 57
Greece, 20, 44, 86
Growth:
    adolescent spurt in, 86–87
    Chinese children and, 88
    Farm Study and, 85–86
    meat and dairy products and, 87–
        88
    myth concerning, 83–88
Grundy, Dr. Scott, 46

Haas, Ellen, 140
*Handbook of Pest Management in Ag-
    riculture*, 126
Hardee's, 52
Hard Rock Cafe, 133
Harper's, 90
Hart, Dr. Ronald, 124, 174, 178
Harvard University, xxvii, 34, 72, 184
    breast cancer study at, xxiii
    Center for Risk Analysis, 191
    colon cancer study at, 57
Haskell, Dr. William, 46
Havala, Suzanne, 78, 171
Hawkins, Anthony, 181
Health, 21
    instinct and, 146
Health, 57
Health hype, combating, 120

Health Star, Guidelines for Health
        School Meal Planning,
        148–49
Heart attacks:
    cholesterol level at time of, 7–8
    hydrogenated fat and, 18
    obesity and, 25
    statistics on, xx
    three generations of prevention of,
        13–14
    Western diet and, 4
Heart Disease and High Cholesterol
    (Conti), 22
Heart Failure (Moore), 97
Heart Healthy Lessons for Children,
    147–48
Heart Smart, 146–47
Hearty School Lunch Program, 148–
    149
Hegsted, Dr. Mark, 65
Helsinki Heart Study, 96–97
Hershey Golden Almond bar, 92
Heslin, Jo-Ann, 70
High-density lipoprotein (HDL), 14–
    15
    saturated fat and, 18
High-fat foods:
    condiments, 92–93
    dairy, 91
    eggs, 91
    hidden, 89–90
    invisible fat, 92
    meat, 90
    myth of obviousness of, 89–94
    snacks, 93–94
    at the White House, 89–90
High Road to Health, The (Wagner
        and Spade), 200
Hiroshima nuclear explosion, xxiii
Hodgkinson, Neville, 11
Holman, Dr. R. L., 155
Hong Kong, 164
Honson, Bob, 145
How to Read the New Food Label,
    122
Huff, Andrea, 148
Hugo, Victor, xxi
Hulley, Dr. Stephen, 189
Human growth hormone, 24
Hummus, 230
Hurley, Jane, 114
Hybrid fruits and vegetables, 111
Hydrogenated fat, 18, 94
Hypertension, xxiv, xxviii, 5, 6, 11, 108

Ideal diet, 42, 101–9, 179
  cold turkey change to, 102
  fiber and, 106–7
  getting started, 128–32
    "Dr. Attwood's Guidelines," 128–129
    "family plan" and, 131–32
    four stages and, 130
    "quiet cooking" and, 131
  nonvitamin and nonmineral ingredients, 107–8
  potassium-sodium ratio and, 108–9
  shopping for, *see* Shopping primer for low-fat foods
  transition to, 102–3
    Stage 1, 103
    Stage 2, 103–4
    Stage 3, 104
    Stage 4, 105, 108–9
  vegetables and, 105–6
Improvement in children's diets, myth of, 50–54
  fat habit returns, 51–52
  fat rampage, 52–53
  high-fat snacks, 53–54
  presidential burger, 53
  race for children's taste buds, 50–51
Inactivity, 5
India, 81
Indoles, 107
Information Resources' InfoScan, 114–115
Inge, W. R., xxxii
International high-fat life-style, 162–71
  in Africa, 169
  in China, 164–66
  in England, 166–67
  in Finland, 168
  in Hong Kong, 164
  in Italy, 167–68
  in Japan, 163–64
  milk and dairy products and, 170–171
  in Singapore, 165
  in South America, 168–69
  in Taiwan, 164
International Journal of Cardiology, 167
Iron, 57–58, 61
Iron-deficiency anemia, 65
Isothiocyanate, 107
Israel, 6, 86

Italian restaurants, 134
Italy, xxiii, 6, 20, 44, 167–68

Jackson, Richard J., 126
Jaeger, Jane, 183
Japan, xxii, 6, 8, 9, 19, 65, 81, 105, 163–64, 185, 187–88
"Jelly-bean effect," 41
Johns Hopkins Complete Guide for Preventing and Reversing Heart Disease, 87
Johns Hopkins University School of Medicine, 87, 162, 170
Johns Hopkins Young Adult Study, 156, 188–89
Johnson, Lyndon, 25
Johnson, Dr. Samuel, 62
Johnson, Suzanne Bennett, 189–90
Jones, Dr. Peter, 44, 133
Journal of Cardiopulmonary Rehabilitation, 46–47
Journal of the American College of Nutrition, 185
Journal of the American Dietetic Associations, 84, 155
Journal of the American Medical Association, 189
Journal of the National Cancer Institute, xxiii

Kashani, Dr. I. A., 164
Kaye, Dr. Freddie, 22
Kellogg's Product 19, 74, 75
Kennedy, John F., xxvii, 25
Kennedy, Robert, xxxi
Kentucky Fried Chicken, 51, 52, 165
Kessler, Dr. David, 121–22
Ketchup, 93
Kimberton Waldorf School, 148
Klaper, Dr. Michael, 201
Kleinman, Dr. Ronald E., 159, 170
Knowles, Dr. John, xx
Know Your Body (KYB) Study, 161–162
Knuiman, Dr. J. T., 168
Kolbe, Dr. Lloyd, xx
Konner, Melvin, 29
Koop, Dr. C. Everett, 125
!Kung San bushmen, 40
Kwiterovich, Dr. Peter O., Jr., 87
Kyushu University, 163

La Leche League International, 201
Lancet, 56, 190

Lasagna, Super-Saucy Eggplant, 238–239
Leaf, Dr. Alexander, 174, 177
Leahy, Patrick, 149
Legumes:
    protein from, 56–60
    shopping for, 113
    variety in, 82
Leibowitz, Dr. Sarah, 40
Lichtenberg, G. C., 181
Liebman, Bonnie, 45
Life expectancy, 178, 192
    misinformation about, 182–84
Limited choices, myth of, 78–82
Limonene, 107
Lincoln, Abraham, 36
Lipid panel, 14, 15
Lipoprotein lipase, 32
Little League football, 23–24
Liver, 17
Loews Ventana Canyon Resort, 173
Loma Linda University, 84
London School of Hygiene and Tropical Medicine, 190
London Times Magazine, 11
Longevity, 43
Louise's Fat-Free, 115
Louis Harris poll, 187
Louisiana Department of Public Health, 169
Louisiana Morbidity Report, 169
Louisiana State University, 40, 144, 146, 154, 185–86
Lovastatin, 192
Low-density lipoprotein (LDL), 14
    iron and, 58
    oxidation of, 72
    receptors, 17
Low-Fat Granola, 229
"Lunch at the Waldorf," 148
Lunch recipes, 230–35

McCall's, 7, 192
McCay, Dr. Cleve, 178
McDonald's, 51, 52, 53, 55, 164, 165
McGovern Committee, 43
Malnourishment, 83, 186
Mandell, Dr. Frederick, xxxi
Mangels, Dr. Reed, 59
Manson, Dr. JoAnn, 72
Margarine, 18
Mary Imogene Bassett Research Institute, 191
Mattes, Richard, 38–39

Mayo Clinic, 46, 161, 186
Mead, Margaret, 99
Meat:
    animal-protein risk, 56–57
    "complete" proteins, 58–59
    cruel joke of, 61
    fat and, 60
    growth retardation and, 87–88
    as high-fat food, 90
    myth concerning, 55–61
    popularity of, 57–58
    shopping for, 115–17
    vegetables compared to, 56, 58–59, 60
Meat substitutes, 117–18
M-E-D-I-C-S, 90–94
Mediterraneans, 19–20
Menstruation, xxii–xxiii, 87
Menus, suggested, 217–21
    breakfasts, 218–19
    dinners, 220–21
    lunches, 219–20
Merck & Co., 186
Metabolism, 31, 32–34
Mevacor, 186
Mexican restaurants, 135
Mickey Mantle's Restaurant and Sports Bar, 31
Milk, xxvi–xxvii, 53
    calcium balance and bone density, 65
    coronary artery disease conference and, 177–78
    growth retardation and, 87–88
    as high-fat food, 91
    myth concerning, 62–69
    osteoporosis and, 63–67
    other health hazards from, 63–65
    protein and, 66, 68–69
    saturated fat from, 63, 64, 69, 170–171
    school lunches and, 142
    as source of calcium, 67–68
    as spoiling a perfect diet, 63
Mindell, Dr. Earl, 139
Minerals, 70, 76–77
Minneapolis Star-Tribune, 186
Mirkin, Dr. Gabe, 42–43
Misinformation, 181–93
    chronic unrecognized diseases and, 187–89
    cost-effectiveness of, 190–91
    credible people and, 191–92

Misinformation (*cont.*)
  eating habits of physicians and, 183–85
  of life expectancy, 182–84
  nutritional backlash and, 183–87, 193
  risk of low cholesterol, 187–90
  truthful but misleading, 185–87
Mitchell, Dr. Allen, xxxi
"Mom's Guide to Happy, Low-Fat Kids, A," 70, 79, 132, 197–216
  eating extremes, 206–10
  feeding babies and young children, 200–2
  food-smart family, 210–16
    disagreeing spouse, 212–13
    making the switch, 211–12
    points to remember, 216
    small changes, 214–15
  "New 4 Food Groups," 198–200
  other people's opinions, 204–6
  out in the world, 203–4
Monell Chemical Senses Center, 38
Monounsaturated fatty acids, 18–19, 20, 34, 113
Moore, T. J., 97
Moran, Victoria, 70, 79, 132, 197–221
Moroccans, 20
Mr. Phipps Pretzel Chips, 114
"Mud" Cookies, 251–52
Muffins:
  Applesauce, 244
  Banana-Oat, 246
Multiple Risk Factor Intervention Trial (MRFIT), 96–97, 188
Multivitamin supplements, 76
Muscatine, Iowa, study, 157–58
Must, Dr. Aviva, 25
Mustard, 93
Mutual of Omaha, 176
Mycoskie, Pam, 160

Nabisco, 114
Nader, Dr. P. R., 164
National Academy of Sciences (NAS), 43, 143
  on animal protein, 56–57
  Committee on Diet and Health, xxi
  Food and Nutrition Board, 47
  on pesticides, 123, 126
  potassium-sodium ratio and, 108
National Beef Industry Council, xxvi, 57, 86, 87

National Cancer Institute (NCI), xxi, 45, 107, 125
  vitamin supplements and, 71–73
National Center for Health Statistics, 85, 159, 182, 184
National Center for Toxicological Research, 124, 178
National Cholesterol Education Program (NCEP), 8, 155
  Adult and Child Treatment Panels, 45, 46, 47
  dietary guidelines of, xxv, xxvi, 43, 46
  heart-disease risk and, 9–10
National Dairy Council, xxvi, xxvii, 62, 68, 86, 87
National Heart, Lung and Blood Institute, 155, 187, 188
National Institute of Environmental Health Sciences Center, 125
National Institutes of Health (NIH), xxiv, xxvii, 103, 155
  cholesterol guidelines of, 5, 12, 13, 43, 156–60, 171, 172, 175–77
  growth retardation and, 83, 86
  school lunches and, 141
National Research Council, 59
National School Lunch Act, 150
National University Hospital in Singapore, 165
Natow, Dr. Annette B., 70
Nestle, Dr. Marion, 43, 46, 111
New American Diet, The (Conner), 29
New England Journal of Medicine, 23, 63, 186
Newman, Dr. Thomas, 189
Newmark, Jane L., 147
Newsweek, 140, 145
New York Times, The, 42, 66, 114, 125, 140, 163, 164, 170, 176, 186
New York University, xxvii, 43, 46, 111
Niacin, 74
Nixon, Richard, 25
Nolen, Dr. William, 191–92
Nonstick cookware, 113–14, 119
Northern Ireland, 4, 168
Northwestern University Medical School, 160
Norway, 43, 190–91
NPD Group, 42
NutriClean, 126
Nutrition Action Healthletter, 65, 80, 115, 134

Nutritional density, 105–6
Nutritional Education and Training (NET), 143, 150
Nutritional extravagance, diseases of, xxviii–xxix
"Nutritional terrorism," 170
Nutrition Labeling and Education Act of 1990, 120–21

Oat bran, 19, 81–82, 93
Oats, 81–82
Obesity, xxviii, 11, 19, 64–65
  adult weight gain, 25–26
  after-school habits and, 22
  calories and, 32–34
  in China, 166
  dealing with, 207–8
  as earliest visible sign of poor health, 21
  emotional issues and, 207–8
  exercise and, 31–32
  as family affair, 26–29
  fat storage and, 34
  football and, 23–24
  growing out of, 24–26
  increasing incidence of childhood, 26
  during the last half-century, 30–31
  myth concerning, 21–35
  risk of early, 35
  "well-fed" look, 23
"Official" guidelines, xxiv–xxviii
Oils, 18, 19
Olive oil, 18, 19, 20
Olivetti, 6
Omae, Dr. Teruo, 163–64
Oparil, Dr. Suzanne, xxiv, 3, 26
Opinions of others, 204–6
Oreos, 94
Ornish, Dr. Dean, 34, 44, 46–47, 89–90, 102, 158, 174, 176
Oschner, Dr. Alton, 87
Oski, Dr. Frank, xxx–xxxi, 62, 170
Osteoporosis, 63–67, 178
Otsego County, New York, 159
Oven Fries, 236
Oxford University, 165
Oxidation, 72

Paleolithic Prescription, The (Eaton et al.), 29–30
Palm oil, 93–94
Palumbo, Dr. P. J., 186
Pancakes, Banana, 225–26

Pantothenic acid, 76
Parents' Nutrition Bible (Mindell), 139
"Partially hydrogenated," 18
Pasta, 112, 134
Pasta Salad, 231
Pathobiological Determinants of Atherosclerosis in Youth (PDAY) Research Group, 155
Pawtucket Heart Health Program, 162
P-coumaric acid, 107
Peanut butter, 18
Peanut-Butter Stretchers, 232
Pearson, Dr. Thomas, 19
Peas, 113
Pediatric Alert, xxxi
Pediatric Nutrition Handbook, 13
Pediatrics, 85
Periactin, 24
Pesticides, 122–26
Pesticides in the Diets of Infants and Children, 123
Phenylketonuria, 158
Physicians' Committee for Responsible Medicine (PCRM), 66, 170, 171, 198
Phytic acid, 108
Phytochemicals, 73, 107–8
Phytosterols, 107
Piccadilly Cafeterias, 53
Picky eaters, 208–9
Pierce, Sonnet, 222–52
Pimentel, David, 126
Pineapple Upside-Down Cake, 245
Pizza, Vegetable, 240–41
Plaques, 167, 182
Polyunsaturated fatty acids, 18–19, 34
Popcorn, 94
Portable Pediatrician, The (Oski), xxx, 62
Ports, Dr. Thomas A., 174
"Position of the American Dietetic Association: Vegetarian Diets," 171
Post Natural Bran Flakes, 75
Potassium-sodium ratio, 108–9
Potato chips, 114–15
Potato(es):
  -Corn Chowder, 237
  Oven Fries, 236
  Salad, 233–34
Power of Your Plate, The (Barnard), 7, 29, 38
Pregnancy, Children, and the Vegan Diet (Klaper), 201

Presidential burger, 53
Prevention, 187
Preventive Medicine, 184
Princeton School District, 168
Principles and Practice of Pediatrics
      (Oski), xxx
Pritikin, Nathan, 192
Produce, shopping for, 110–12
Prostate cancer, xxii, 56
Protein, 32
   "complete," 58–59
   legumes and, 82
   meat and, *see* Meat
   milk and, 66, 68–69
   vegetable, 56, 58–59, 60
Public Health Service, 11
Public Voice for Food and Health Pol-
      icy, 140, 150
Pyridoxine, 74–75

Questran, 13–14
"Quiet cooking," 131

Recipes, 222–52
   breakfast, 223–29
   dessert and bread, 243–52
   lunch, 230–35
   supper, 236–42
Recommended Dietary Allowances
      (RDAs) for protein, 59
Red wine, 19
"Refried" Beans, 237–38
Rensi, Edward, 53
Restaurant food, *see* Eating out
Riboflavin, 74, 80, 171
Rice, 112
Rifkin, Jeremy, 61
Rifkind, Dr. Basil, 155, 174
Road to Wellville, The (Boyle), 55
Roberts, Dr. William, 5
Roberts, Michael, 193
Rockefeller University, 40
Rocky Mountain News, 186
Root-beer milk, 142

Safflower oil, 18
St. Paul's School, 16
Salad bars, 136
Salad Dressing, Veggie, 235
Salt, 93
Sanmarco, Dr. Miguel E., 174
Saturated fat, xxvi–xxviii, 5, 34, 44, 46
   controlling high cholesterol levels
      and, 16–19

in dairy products, 63, 64, 69, 91,
      170–71
   described, 18–19
   invisible, 92
   in meat, 57, 60, 61, 90
   misinformation about, *see*
      Misinformation
   in vegetable oil, 113
Sauces, 93
Schaefer, Dr. Ernst, 46
Scheib, Walter S., III, 90
School lunch program, 139–50
   deep frying and, 140–41
   health-conscious administrators,
      148–49
   high-fat, 143
      saving money and, 143–44
   legislation and, 149–50
   lunches from home versus, 203–4
   LUNCHPOWER! program, 146–47
   misinformation about, 141–42
   model, 147–48
   root-beer milk, 142
   success stories, 145–46
   USDA and, 139–44, 148–50
Schuette, Cathy, 148
Schweitzer, Dr. Albert, 41
Science, 66
Scotland, xxii, 4, 168
Seventh-Day Adventists, xxii, xxviii, 7,
      84
Shaw, George Bernard, xxxi
Shellfish, 115, 116
Shintani, Dr. Terry, 31
Shipley, Jeanette, 148
Shopping primer for low-fat foods,
      110–27
   beans and peas, 113
   canola oil, 113
   dairy, 118
   health-hype and, 120
   meat and fish, 115–17
   meat substitutes, 117–18
   nonstick cookware, 113–14,
      119
   one-stop shopping, 120
   pesticides and, 122–23
      exaggerated risk of, 123–26
   produce, 110–12
      cleaning, 126–27
   recent sales growth, 110
   snacks, 114–15
   tips for, 119
   updated food labels and, 120–22

Shostak, Marjorie, 29–30
Shrimp, 17
Silent Spring (Carson), 124
Simplesse, 37
Singapore, 20, 165
Singer, Dr. Dorothy, 22
Smith, E. O., 39
Smoking, 5, 6, 7, 45, 48, 86, 162
Smoothies, Fruit-Juice, 227
Snack Food, 53
Snacks:
    high-fat, 53–54, 93–94
    low-fat, 94
    shopping for, 114–15
SnackWell's Cracked Pepper Crackers, 114
SnackWell's Wheat Crackers, 114
Sodium, 93
    potassium-sodium ratio, 108–9
Soup:
    Potato-Corn Chowder, 237
    Tomato-Vegetable, 234–35
South Africa, 169
South America, xxi, 168–69
Soybean oil, 18
Soybeans, 56, 117, 118
Spade, Ariane, 200
Spinach, 111
Spock, Dr. Benjamin, vii–x, 23, 37–38, 170
Stanford University, 46, 183
Starc, Dr. Thomas, 22
Stary, Dr. H. C., 155
Stewart, Dr. Kerry, 162
Stone Age:
    diet during, 30
    fat-craving genes from, 39–40
Strawberry:
    Fruit Shake, Banana-, 228
    "Ice Cream," 225
Stringer, Dr. Bobby, 31
Stroke, xxiv, xxviii, 11, 25
Substance abuse, economic cost of, 48
Suicide, 187–88
Sunflower-seed oil, 18
Super-Saucy Eggplant Lasagna, 238–239
Supper recipes, 236–42
Sweden, 43, 65
Sweet potato, 80
"Sweets," 92
"Sweet taste," 37

Taiwan, 164
Taming of the Shrew, The, 78
Taste buds, 36–37
Taxes on fat, 48–49
Taylor, Jerry, 124
T.G.I. Friday's, 133
Thermogenesis, 31
Thiamin, 74
Time, 50, 52
Token reductions of dietary fat, 41–49
    consumer choice and, 46–47
    fears of discouraging the public and, 43–49
    NCEP and, 46, 47
    recommended fat keeps falling, 43–44
    tax on fat and, 48–49
    timid doctors and, 45
    timid government agencies and, 45
    trimming the fat, 42–43
Tomato sauce, 93
Tomato-Vegetable Soup, 234–35
Total Corn Flakes, 74, 75
Total Raisin Bran, 74
Total Wheat Flakes, 74
Trans fatty acids, 18
Treatment approach of Western medicine, xxiv–xxv
Triglycerides, 14–15
Tufts University, xxvii, 25, 26, 46, 71, 75
Tufts University Diet & Nutrition Letter, 186
Turkey, 115, 116
Turks, 86
TV watching, 22
    commercials and, 202
Twain, Mark, 101, 181

UCLA, 178
United Nations, 124
    Food and Agriculture Organization, 164–65
U.S. Department of Agriculture (USDA), xxix, 79, 80
    Food Guide Pyramid, 73, 101
    four food groups of, 141–42
    school lunch programs and, 139–144, 148–50
U.S. Senate Agriculture Committee, xxix, 149
U.S. Senate Select Committee on Nutrition and Human Needs, 43

United States Preventive Services Task Force, 11
University of California at Berkeley, 125
University of California at Berkeley Wellness Letter, 63, 115
University of California at San Diego Department of Community and Family Medicine, 84
University of California at San Francisco, 189
University of Florida, 189
University of Illinois Child Development Laboratory, 37
University of Iowa, 157
  Department of Preventive Medicine and Environmental Health, 27
University of Minnesota, 146, 186
University of Naples, 6
University of Southern California, 46
University of Texas Lifetime Health Letter, 80
University of Troms, 190
University of Turku, 168
U.S. News & World Report, 111
USA Today, 90
USDA/FNS/CND, 143

Van Camp, Dr. Steven, 153
Vegetable oils, 17
  shopping for, 113
Vegetable Pizza, 240–41
Vegetables:
  calcium and, 66–68
  cleaning, 126–27
  genetically altered, 81
  pesticides and, 122–26
  protein and, 56, 58–59, 60
  shopping for, 110–12
  Stage 4 diet and, 105–6
  variety in, 79–80, 82, 199
  vitamins, minerals, and, 70–77
Vegetable Soup, Tomato-, 234–35
Vegetarian Chili, 242
Vegetarian Journal, 59
Vegetarians, xxii, xxviii, 7, 9, 15, 28, 73–74
  myth of growth retardation in, 83–88
Veggie Salad Dressing, 235
Venezuela, 168–69
Vice, Lauren, 89
Viikari, Dr. J., 168

Virmani, Dr. Renu, 174
Vitamins:
  A, 71, 80, 81
  B-complex, 73–76, 80, 105
  C, 71, 72–73, 80, 81, 111
  D, 72
  E, 72–73
  K, 73
  misinformation about, 185–86
  myth concerning, 70–76
  supplements of, 71–73

Wagner, Lindsay, 200
Walford, Dr. Roy, 178
Waller, Robert James, 131
Wall Street Journal, 52, 121, 170, 186
Walnuts, 19
Walsh, Dr. Judith, 191
Warshaw, Hope, 138
Washington Post, The, 53
Weaver Light, 94
Weidman, Dr. William, 46
Weisburger, Dr. John, xxiii
We Live Too Short and Die Too Long (Bortz), 184
"Well-fed" look, 23
Wendy's, 52, 183
Western Dairyfarmers' Association, 142
Whitaker, Robert C., 145, 146
Whitford Corporation, 114
Whole grains, 81–82
Wholesome and Hearty Foods, 104, 117, 134
Wild Game, 17, 30
Willett, Dr. Walter, xxiii, 18, 57
Wittrock, Donna, 142
Womanly Art of Breastfeeding, The (La Leche League), 201
Woolf, Dr. Steven, 11
Woolf, Virginia, 151
Woolley, Dr. Bruce, 24
World Health Organization, 124
Wynder, Dr. Ernest L., 21, 44, 47, 86, 87, 162–63, 168, 174, 177

Yale University Family Television Research and Consultation Center, 22
Yankee Stadium, 31
York, David, 40
Young children, feeding, 200–2